22
So Young
Why Did He Die?

by

Barbara Kimbley

authorHOUSE™

1663 LIBERTY DRIVE, SUITE 200
BLOOMINGTON, INDIANA 47403
(800) 839-8640
WWW.AUTHORHOUSE.COM

First published by AuthorHouse 12/28/2004

ISBN: 1-4208-1104-5 (sc)

Printed in the United States of America
Bloomington, Indiana

This book is printed on acid-free paper.

Dedicated to my brother, Nicholas who I loved with all my heart and soul. At age 22, he lost the battle with the dreaded and incurable illness, A.I.D.S. He died of hepatic liver failure caused by the disease.

As I gathered stories, comments and thoughts about Nicholas for this book, I was amazed at how many people were supportive. They remembered Nicholas and I immediately, almost 18 years later. People willingly and lovingly added to this story and I am truly grateful.

Acknowledgments

Thank you to my husband, Rich for challenging me every step of the way. You asked the questions that needed to be answered. Thank you for loving my brother, Nickey like your own son. I love you!

Thank you, Rich Jr., my son for accepting my brother, Nickey into our hearts, our homes and our lives. It was difficult for all of us.

Thank you mother, for helping us make lemonade out of lemons in our lives-to see the silver lining in every cloud-to be strong in times of adversity.

Thank you to my sister, for loving me, being my friend and life-long Scrabble partner.

Thank you to my sister-in-law, Chris McClary(Sis) who videotaped 15 minutes of Nickey while he was alive, energetic, funny and lovable. You gave me the most precious gift of all.

Thank you to my brother-in-law and sister-in-law, Bill and Dianne Kimbley for opening your hearts and home to us and taking the trip to the cabin in Arietta,

N.Y. after Nickey died so we could grieve together as a family.

Thank you, Kathy Rooney for helping me insert the photos and encouraging me to write this story. When I said,"I only have 10 Microsoft pages".

You said, "Barbara, you can do it" "Don't give up". "It's a great story!"

Thank you Gee-Gee for the time you spent talking to me about the conversations you had with Nick. I appreciate your input in the story.

Thank you -Nassau County Medical Center, East Meadow, Long Island, New York, for having a team of nurses, doctors and staff who were knowledgeable,nurturing and caring in my brothers final days of his short life.

Thank you to the Priests of St. Malachys Church and St. Gregorys Church and all the churches worldwide for your continued prayers.

Thank you Boston Bill Bonick for providing me an E computer so I can finish this book and start on my next one. You still owe me lunch and a drink or are we even now?

Thank you Bob T .for providing the Microsoft 2000 program so I could edit this book. You said, you'd be the first one to buy my book? Thanks for your continuous prayers.

Thank you to all my J.C. Penney associates and friends for being there through the happy and sad times.

You helped me get through a tragic time and climb an insurmountable mountain.

Thank you to my neighbors and friends for listening and encouraging me to write this book, especially when I was feeling discouraged.

Thank you to all my family and friends for being there when I needed you the most. You gave me love, faith and strength to face the next day.

A letter written, November 10, 1986 in Nickey's own words...This is a message to the world-19 days before he died. He died November 29,1986.

I'm 22 years old and I caught a fatal disease. And I'm scared. I'm out of work I'm going to miss everybody I don't know how long I have to live. And I hope everybody forgives me for what I did years ago.

I straightened my life 3 ½ years ago and now it is shot. I just have to live day by day.

My back is killing me, too. I had a piece of bone taken out of my back on Friday. My eyes are bloodshot.

I was shocked when I heard I had this disease. I felt like killing myself in the hospital. I was shocked. I had someone watching outside the door so I couldn't kill myself.

I love my mother and I hope she doesn't drink too much and I want her to do good. I hope she'll be alright when I'm gone.

I love my sister Barbara and I love Richie. And, I love Richie Jr. They have been my family for the past several years.

I worked and I have a lot of good friends and I thank them for everything they've done for me while I was out of work and in the hospital-the cards and visits-candy, cookies, soda.

I love Andrea and I thank her for everything. I'm sorry I was so sick.

I used to drink and smoke and I quit then, I got sick. I started these two evils at a young age, about 12 years old.

My father was an alcoholic. He died at age 44 of cirrhosis of the liver.

I had a bad life coming from a bad home. I took to the streets at a young age. My security were my friends.

I quit school at age 13-finished grammar school and that's the extent of my education.

I like to watch TV. I don't read much-I guess cause I really don't know how. I do pick up Newsday every now and then.

People call me "street-wise". Nobody can pull anything over on me. I see right through them. After all, I grew up in lower Manhattan on the streets. I saw everything - everything from drugs, to robberies to murders. One day, my buddy and I were standing on a street corner and some guy came up to us, opened up his trench coat and blew my buddy away with a shotgun. I know people from all walks of life.

I'm a friendly person. I talk to people and I learn about them. At first, I can be shy but, once I know someone, I talk to them.

I used to be paranoid when I came to live on Long Island. I couldn't believe the difference from the city to the Island. I walked to the deli in Wantagh, early in the evening and there were no people on the streets. It felt so strange. I'm used to people all over in the city at all times of day and night.

When I was a little boy, I wanted to grow up and be a garbage collector. At my job, I used to pick up garbage. I didn't make much money but I did something I always wanted to do. It turned out, it really wasn't for me- so, then I got a stock boy job.

In life, I could make something out of nothing. I could pick up a sewing machine, fix it and sell it and make a few bucks out of something that was thrown in the garbage.

SHORTLY AFTER MIDNIGHT

The day I called on Jesus
Was the day my life was changed
It was shortly after midnight
No one heard me call His name
I was twenty-two and trying
Hard to hold onto my life
In a world I sold my soul to for a title and a price
How do I sing of the trip I took
Through the days and the sins of my past
Looking through eyes that no longer were mine
To be seen and forgiven at last
I remember a feeling of calmness
That washed over all the fears in my mind
A feeling of warmth and protection
That existed before there was time
I reached out and saw the angel of light
And I knew that I wasn't alone
And I knew that somewhere high above me
Was my Father, my Lord, and my Home
how do I sing of the love that He gave
When He died for the sins of my past
I have been freed; I am no longer a trapped
in an uncertain world
I am His, I am forgiven at Last.

UNKNOWN

Nickey's Childhood

On January 22,1964, in Lincoln Hospital, South Bronx, NY, my brother Nicholas Mike was born. A bouncing baby boy with brown hair, big brown eyes and an olive complexion. My mother Ethel was overprotective and his father, Mike was an epileptic and violent alcoholic. He had many episodes where he went into statuesque positions and also banged his head on the wooden floor, screaming," I'm coming home daddy". It was a frightening scene for children to see.

Nicholas had two sisters, Lana and Barbara. Lana, the oldest sister was already married and had one baby at the time. She offered to take Nickey several times, but my mother refused her offers. Lana now is a mother of four grown children and five grandchildren. Her oldest son, Frank died at age 36, leaving his beloved wife and son, Sean and stepson, Randy here on Earth. Dennis 36 lives in Orlando, Florida. Jennifer, Lana's daughter now 31 years old , is the mother of three children, Anthony, Cheito and Alex. Russell is twenty-one years old and is in the Army, stationed in Louisiana.

Barbara was his middle sister who vowed to be there for him always. Barbara and Nicholas were five years apart. Barbara assumed the surrogate mother role at a very young age; loving and nurturing her brother-changing his diapers, feeding him, dressing him and later teaching him.

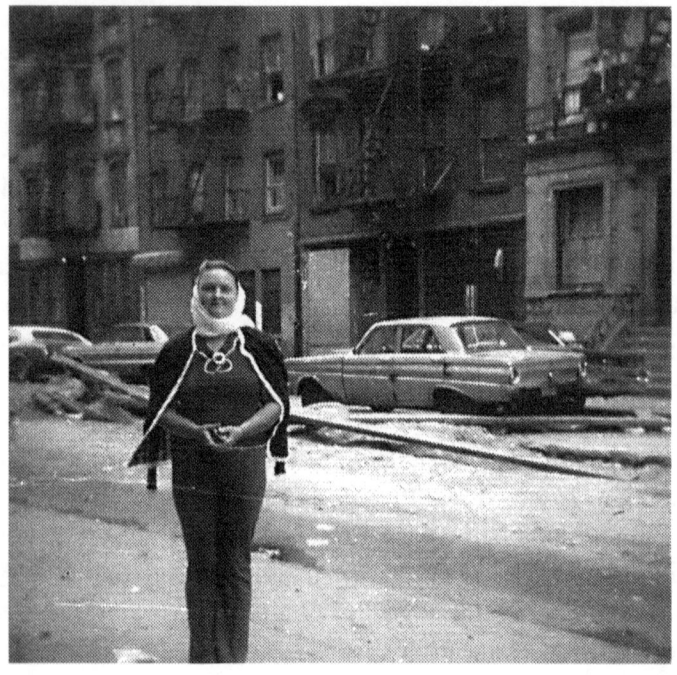

Nickey's Mother Ethel East 13th St. New York City

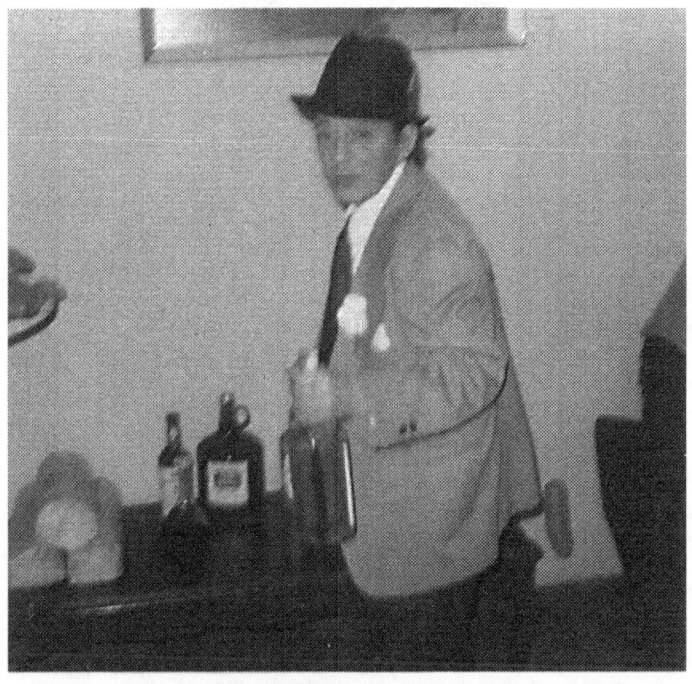

Nick's Father Mike New York City

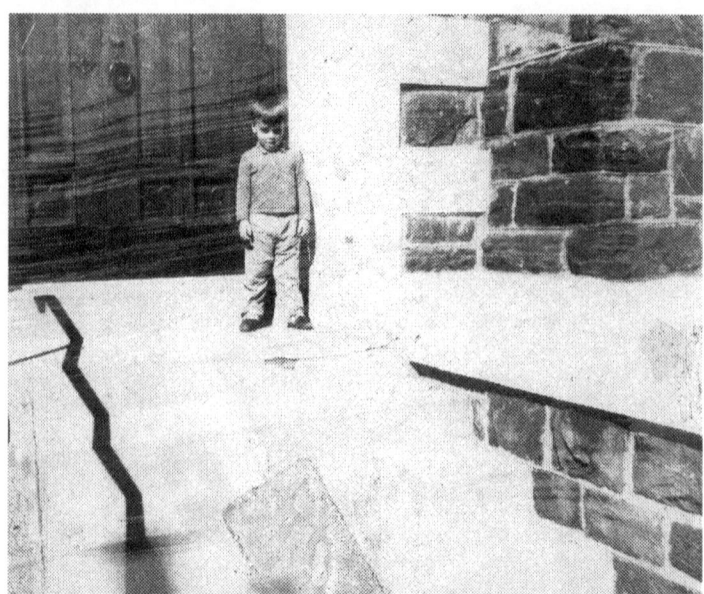

This is a picture of Nickey at Barbara's Holy Communion, Saint Mary's Church Bronx New York.

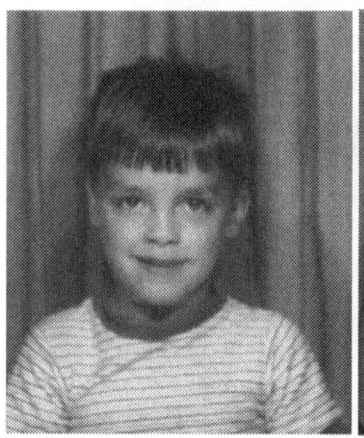

Nickey 5 years old

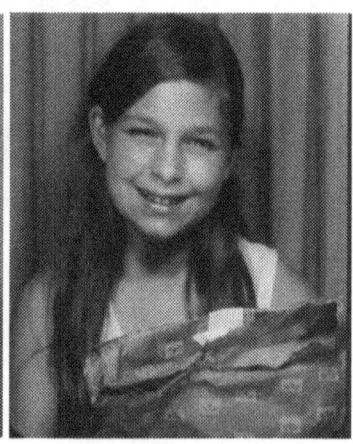

Barbara 10 Years old

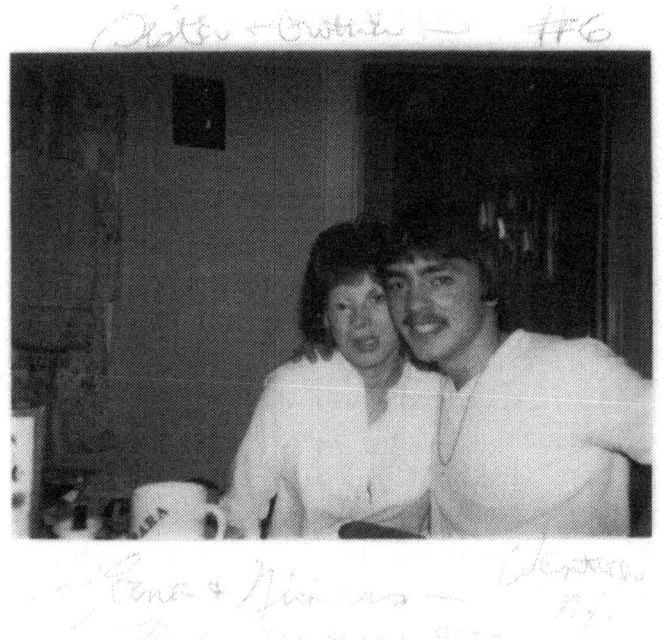

Lana & Nick

In their early years Barbara and Nickey loved to play teacher and student but unfortunately, due to a dysfunctional environment, Barbara moved away at a very young age. Barbara was passed around to many different relatives, leaving Nicholas to fend for himself and he eventually quit school.

Nickey is remembered by Sister Theresa, a nun from the Catholic Workers Home, as being a nice but troubled kid. At the time his father was dying he would ride his bicycle up and down the streets in front of the Catholic Worker Home. He seemed lost and sad and desperately in need of help. A man who resided at the home approached Sister Theresa on behalf of Nickey,

5

which shortly thereafter opened the door for Nickey at the home.

Sister Renee, a Dominican teacher at the home, helped to get Nickey back in school and continued to help him with his studies. Nickey was a likable kid with a bad break in life.

Cathy C., a worker (now a teacher in Minnesota) remembers Nickey coming to the Catholic Worker's Home in NYC due to a very upsetting home life. He was emotionally distressed. His mother, Ethel, was a nervous, insecure and fearful woman. Nickey and his parents would frequently fight.

Nickey and his father have threatened each other with knives, on more than one occasion. There was constant violence and fighting in the home between Nickey and his parents.

Nick was about 11 years old when Cathy C. met him. He was the only child that lived there among adults. He always wanted to help and to please. He wanted to be accepted.

Nickey was enrolled in school and Cathy C. assisted him with his homework. He was smart but always distracted. He was a sweet boy and Cathy was very fond of him.

Nickey Missed His Mother.

Nickey moved back home and trouble started again. The workers helped him get into Dobbs Ferry Children's Village, Yorktown, NY This was a home for children from dysfunctional families and emotionally disturbed children.

Nick stayed there awhile. Rich and I visited him and brought him clothes, sneakers, candy and cookies.

Nickey missed his mother and his father was very sick. He ran away from Dobbs Ferry and back home. He ended up on the streets of NYC.

Rich and I offered to take him to live with us but my mother refused our offer. She did not want to be alone with her dying husband.

After his father died at age 44, of cirrhosis of the liver Nickey introduced his mother to Sister Theresa and she was offered to live there since she needed a place to stay. Sister Theresa continues to be friends with my mother helping her with food, money, prayers and a place to visit. . Nickey ran away from the Catholic Workers Home, after his father died. Nicholas found life on the streets of NYC living a life of drugs and crime. He quit school again.

He learned the hard knocks of life on the streets. His friends taught him to speak Spanish, which he learned fluently without classroom instruction. He never knew where his next meal was coming from or where he would sleep. He often slept on a park bench or an alleyway in Spanish Harlem, so strung out on drugs, not caring about anything.

Our mother turned to alcohol and the streets to ease her pain and suffering. Her entire life was traumatic and tragic so as a result our lives followed the pattern of our mother's. Ethel was one of eleven children, seven girls and four boys. She left home at a very young age. First living in Catholic homes then moving on her own as a teenager. Nicholas ended up in prison several times. Sometimes it was better to be in prison, he learned because you knew you were getting fed and you had a place to sleep.

My cousin Gee Gee had a conversation with Nick once about his prison experience. Nick had a bad drug habit and he got in trouble with the law. Nick hired a lawyer and paid him a lot of money. The lawyer went to court with Nick to represent him but he did not say anything to help him. Nick said, "I could have defended myself better".

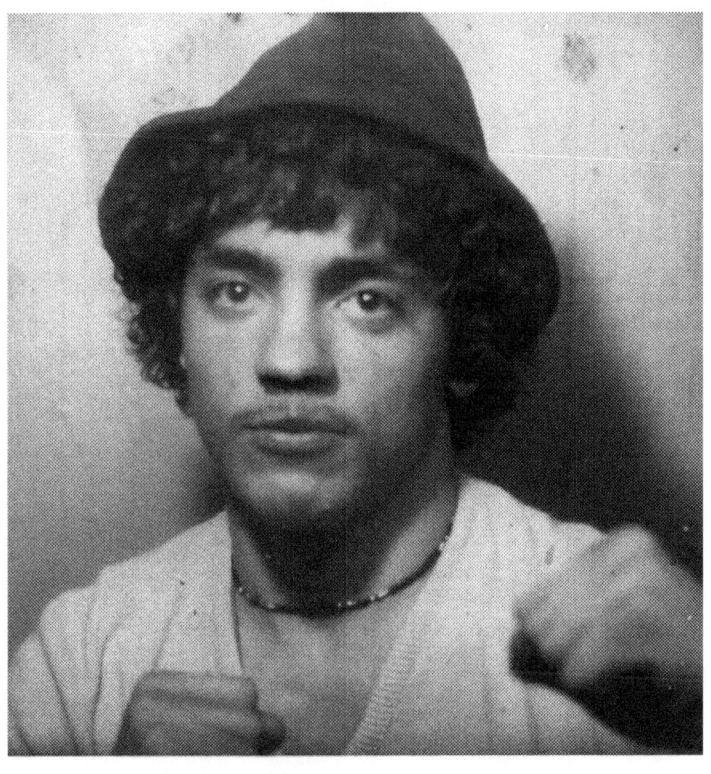

Nickey's Rikers Island Experience

The judge sent Nick to Rikers Island, which is located between the Bronx and Queens, NY-a very hard-core prison. He was sentenced to serve 7 months and 17 years probation. He should have never been sent there. Very sad-traumatic experience.

Cell Blocks

Gee Gee said, Nicks first day in prison, a prisoner asked Nick," WHAT SIZE SHOE DO YOU WEAR"? Nick said, "I WEAR YOUR SIZE"! The prisoner and Nick had a big fight- a violent fight. Nick had to stand up for his rights and show he was not afraid. The prisoner never bothered him again.

Nick lived in a 10 ft. long, 6 ft. wide cell with no toilet. You had to hold it in until the guard unlocked your cell and let you use the bathroom.

When Nick went to breakfast, lunch or dinner, the prisoners would bother him all the time. There were times when he would sit in the cell and not eat because he did not want to be bothered. Sometimes, he would starve himself.

Nick would sit in his cell and cry all day long.

Nick told Gee Gee, "When a man is on Rikers Island, the man knows who his friends are." Nick said, my mother visited me everyday.

Gee Gee said, Nick was a hard man but an honest man with himself. Gee Gee remembers one time, Nick took $1.00 out of his car and never put it back. Nick said he needed the dollar. Gee Gee said," the Meek are the Mighty." Nick, if you need the $1 that bad, keep it!"

Nick had a hard life. Nick's father was a horrible alcoholic and his mother a lost soul. Nick never had a chance.

Nick had a hard time talking to people. He did not trust too many people. Nick said it was easy to talk to GeeGee. He liked GeeGee.

GeeGee said ,I wish Nick were here today to talk to. Nick would take away some of my loneliness and give me some of his strength. You felt better after talking to Nick. He was strong and charismatic. GeeGee said, "I liked Nick." "He just never had a chance in life."

Barbara And BarbaraJo Visit Nickey At Rikers Island

In the Fall or Winter of 1982, Barbara Jo picked me up at my house in Wantagh to drive to Rikers Island. She thought it was going to be like a prison in Nassau County on Old Country Road. She asked her dad (who was a truck driver all his life) for directions to Rikers Island.

Then, we drove in her Toyota down a very guarded road, where a cop was waving for everyone to park in the parking lot and get on the bus.

We boarded a school bus, in which we were the only two minorities. We dressed up and we stood out. The bus was full of adults and screaming kids, who all seemed to be from the inner city.

The bus took us over a long bridge. We got off the bus and walked to the main building. It gave us both an eerie feeling, like a vision of Alcatraz from the movies.

We walked in the main building and we were wanded and searched. Our pocketbooks and possessions were carefully checked. We signed in to see Nickey. We sat down in a waiting room and waited a long time. We watched families visit prisoners and give them gifts.

After awhile, BarbaraJo got up and approached the attendant. She asked, "How much longer do we have to wait to see Nickey?"

The attendant said, Nickey already had a visitor today, which was his mother and only one visitor is allowed daily.

Barbara Jo and I left feeling sad and depressed, not knowing if Nickey would be told we attempted to see him.

Nickey Visited Us
On Long Island

After being released from prison, Nick began to visit us on Wantagh, L.I. We enjoyed having him around.

I remember Nickey being amazed at how there were no people walking on the streets. He was used to the noisy and busy life of NYC...the city that never sleeps...Long Island was much quieter.

Lee and Rommie, our dear family friends became very fond of Nickey. When Nickey visited he would organize their cabinets, rearrange the furniture, paint the bathroom and keep Lee company. Lee and Nickey cooked and baked together.

This brings me to the time, etched in my memory and in my heart, when Lee gave Nickey her favorite cake recipe, the Sweetheart Cake with Orange Icing.

Lee guided Nickey to bake a surprise birthday cake for me, which he did with love and great joy.

It was a sweetheart cake from scratch. The homemade icing was made with oranges and lemons and confectionery sugar.

Another surprise awaited me. I came home from a trying day at work and my sister, Lana was there. She and her baby son, Russell drove up from Florida to celebrate my birthday. It was a memorable day.

One day, Lee dressed Nickey up in a navy blue suit, white dress shirt and tie and she said she had a surprise for him.

They took a train into NYC. Lee treated Nickey to a delicious dinner at Sardis restaurant. Then they went to Barnum and Bailey Circus at Madison Square Garden.

Nickey was so excited. Lee and Nickey had a wonderful time and it did our hearts good to see him so happy.

Lee sold her house, after her husband Rommie died to Jim and Pam K.

We lived there for a short while until we moved to an apartment in Levittown, L.I. Nick continued to visit us. He stayed on weekends. Then....

Rich and I Opened Our Hearts and Home To Nickey

One day, my husband ,Rich and I opened our home and hearts to Nicholas ,not knowing what to expect. He was paranoid and he trusted nobody. He was fearful. And he needed to be loved, nurtured. I hugged him everyday like a daily vitamin, sometimes several times a day. It was a hard road to tread full of sadness and joy. We took on a big responsibility being a young couple, raising a teenage son, ourselves. Eventually, Nicholas felt our love and was very appreciative of the second chance in life. He did a 360 degree turnaround. He changed his life for the better. He completely stopped drugs, criminal activity, cut down on his drinking and smoking cigarettes, found a job at a Major Retail Store which he loved.

He felt proud of himself and his newfound life. He made new friends, and became best friends with our son, Rich Jr. They were tight like brothers; Nicholas being the older brother image. He nurtured and cared for our son and showed him the right path to follow in life by his real life example.

Nickey And Rich Jr. Venture Into NYC

My son, Rich Jr. remembers my husband and I being on vacation to Florida and he and Nick traveling to NYC, knowing they were forbidden to do so.

He and Nickey were talking over breakfast and Nickey said, Hey do you want to go the city with me?

Rich Jr. Recalls taking a long walk to the bus stop, taking the Long Island Railroad into Penn Station. They got off at Penn Station and took a few buses to East 13th Street in Manhattan, Nickey's old neighborhood.

They walked down the street and Nickey was called in every direction…apparently they had a lot of Nicknames for him but Rich does not remember them.

They met up with a guy named Cowboy and a Spanish guy and a few other friends., maybe Tato or Tito…. They hung out and talked in the street for about 45 minutes to an hour.

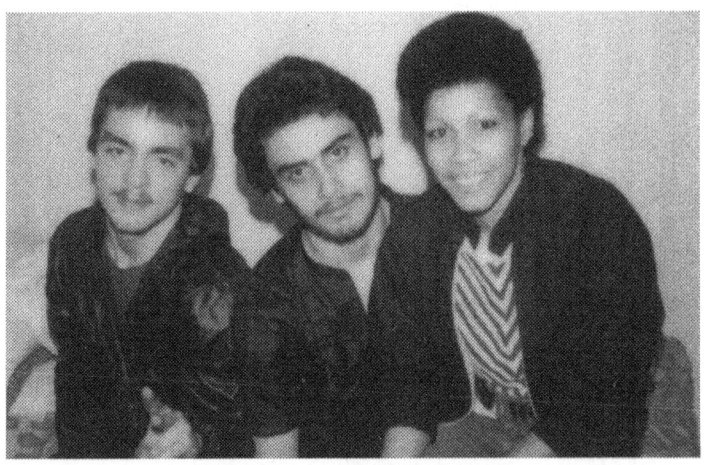

Then they went up on the rooftop (called tar beach) of Nickeys friend's apartment building.

Rich Jr. vividly remembers the pigeons and he was fascinated by their performance. Nickeys friend showed them how the pigeons could fly. He waved a flag in his hand and the pigeons did tricks.

They sat around and had a couple of beers, talked and reminisced about the old days and how Nick's life changed for the better. He got a second chance, living on Long Island with his sister and her family.

They talked about how they climbed down fire escapes and robbed the apartments when people were not home. One day, a resident was home and they got beat up with a baseball bat. Another time, the cops came and caught them and they went to Rikers Island.

They did a lot of partying and needed money for drugs. Some guys had a $400 a day drug habit.

This was the first time Rich Jr. was in New York City in the lower Eastside. He said he felt excited and up for the adventure. Everyone knew Nickey so he felt safe.

Rich and Nick kept their little forbidden adventure a secret for awhile. They did not even visit my mother for fear she would tell us they were there. Eventually we found out about it. We were not happy about it but we were thankful they were safe and unharmed.

Nickey Buys Andrea A Big And Beautiful Garfield

Rich Jr, also, recalls a time Nickey and his girlfriend Andrea took him to the Massapequa Mall. Andrea shopped at one end of the mall and Nickey and Rich shopped at the other end.

Nick wanted to surprise Andrea with something special so he bought her a big and beautiful Garfield stuffed animal .He gave it to Rich to hold.

They stopped for a bite to eat and ice - cream in the food court and guess what?

They walked away from the food court and Rich accidentally left Garfield behind. They walked back to the food court and it was gone.

Nickey was so mad!!! He gave Rich money and demanded he go buy another big and beautiful Garfield stuffed animal for Andrea.

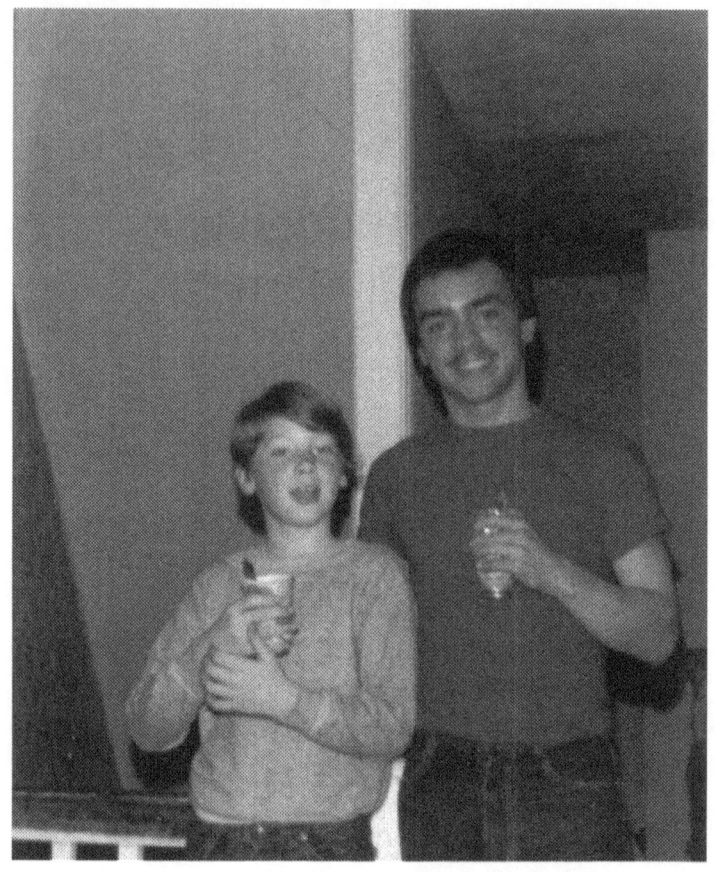

Rich Jr. & Nickey

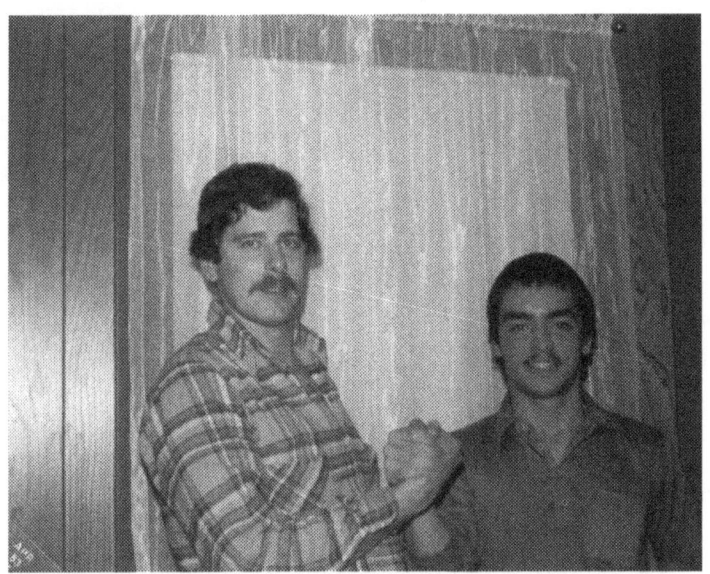

Richard and Nick Wantagh New York

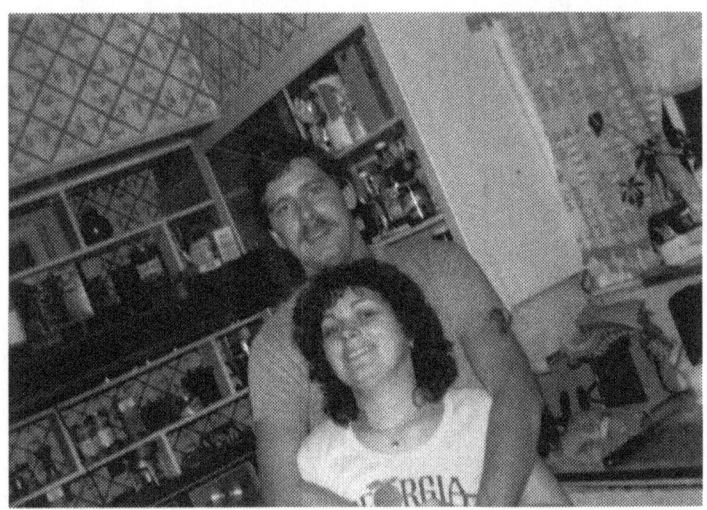

Barbara & Rich

Nickey Runs Away

Out of the clear blue, one day, Nicholas decided to run away from our home, his job and his new life. He took to the streets of NYC again. We were heartbroken. Somehow, we saved his job , hoping and praying he would come to his senses and return home to his new -found life. Well. After crying rivers of tears and phone calls and cajoling, he agreed to come home. Rich picked him up at the Wantagh Railroad station. He looked like hell-extreme weight loss, face drawn, hair messed up, clothes slept in and just lost and forlorn. He was in desperate need of help! The worst part is the drugs got the best of him. He was high on cocaine. My husband had to pour gallons of water and orange juice into him and sit up with him all night.

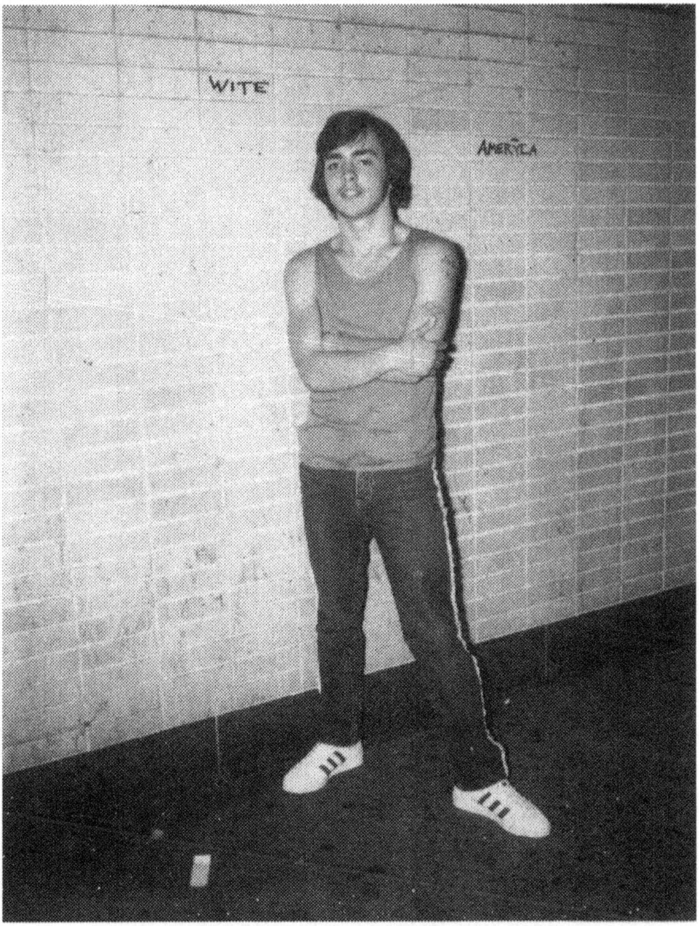

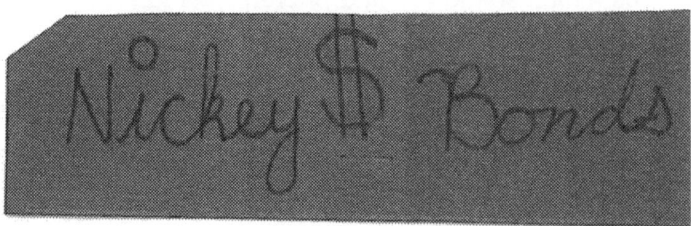

New York Subway (Nick on the run)

"The Last Straw"

We were so hurt, Rich said," this is the last straw". He literally went to the bank and withdrew $1,000. He put the $1,000 on the kitchen table in clear view. He said if Nicholas steals this money then we can wash our hands of this situation and be guilt-free. We have done everything, physically, emotionally and spiritually to help this young man.

Lo and behold, Nicholas never touched the money or anything else that did not belong to him again. He even put a lock on his bedroom door to protect his own hard-earned possessions from thieves in the night. My husband said," Nick, let me ask you a question; Did a lock ever stop you from getting in? "Nick said, "No". "Rich said you need to learn to trust people".   He got on his hands and knees and prayed to God. We prayed together, as we often did. We prayed to God and Virgin Mary.

And we prayed to St. Jude and St. Anthony the following prayers:

Prayer in honor of St. Jude

Through the intercession of St. Jude, cousin of Christ,
May God heed my call for help:

Lord, hear my prayer.
Through the intercession of St. Jude, friend of Christ,
May I always rely upon the loving mercy of God
In all my difficulties;

Lord, hear my prayer.
Through the intercession of St. Jude, apostle of Christ,
May the Holy Spirit listen favorably to my
Urgent prayers and fill me with help:

Lord, hear my prayer.
Through the intercession of St. Jude, martyr of Christ,
May my love of god increase in the midst of troubles:

Lord, hear my prayer.
Through the intercession of St. Jude, priest of Christ,
May the blessings I ask God descend upon me
And remain always:

Lord hear my prayer.

My petition is:

God, St. Jude brought us to the knowledge of your
Holy Name. May our progress in virtue honor His eternal
Glory and May the honor we pay him make us holy.
Through Jesus Christ our Lord. Amen.

Unknown

ST.. ANTHONY
SAINT OF MIRACLES

Holy St. Anthony, reach down from
Heaven and take hold of my hand.
Assure me that I am not alone.
You are known to possess miraculous
Powers and be ever ready to speak
For those in trouble.
Loving and Gentle St. Anthony, reach
down from heaven I implore you and
Assist me in my hour of need. Obtain for me
A renewed life-a second chance.
Dearest St. Anthony, reach down
From heaven and guide me with thy strength.
Plead for me in my needs. And teach me to
Be humbly thankful as you were for all the
bountiful blessings I am to receive.
Amen.
Unknown

He vowed to change his life. He went back to
work, where he was loved and missed. He worked for
an honest living and lived a good life.

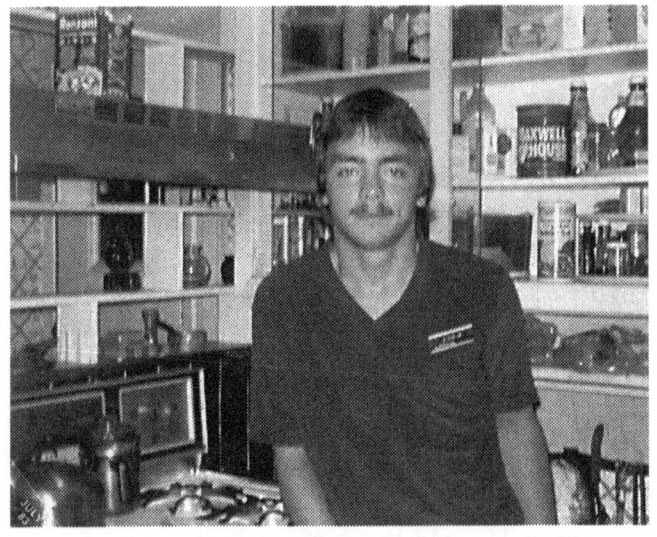

#19   8-19-86

Dear Nicky,
I Really
Love you!
your also
my "Baby"
Love
always
andrea.

Nickey Fell In Love

Nickey dated several girls until he found the one he said he would spend the rest of his life with. Her name was Andrea. He said she reminded him a lot of me, the sister he loved and cherished. They loved each other and they fought like cats and dogs but they were a cute couple. They dreamed of getting married and having a little, Nickey and a little Andrea running around.

Their dreams were shattered when tragedy struck. Nicholas became ill and his life came to a screeching halt.

A.I.D.S. is a dreadful and incurable disease caused by blood transfusions, sharing infected drug needles and promiscuous sex. We are not sure which one took his life. He lived a fast life and he died at the age of 22.

AIDS IN MY OWN WORDS

AIDS affects men, women and children. This disease can affect all races, religions and nationalities. It is a breakdown of the immune system where the white blood cells can no longer fight to survive. One usually dies not of AIDS but of pneumonia, hepatitis or a disease that cannot be fought off because of the weak immune system.

A person can get AIDS from blood transfusions, infected drug needles and promiscuous sex. It is as much a homosexual disease as a heterosexual disease. Saliva has not been proven to cause AIDS. It is not contagious. Casual contact-only in the exchange of blood or semen cannot contract it. It is tested by a simple blood test. Sometimes, a person is diagnosed as an HIV carrier and can live a healthy life, with good nutrition and medication, careful and protected sex.

Back in 1986, there was so little known about AIDS that people died quickly and feared the disease like the plague. Presently, there is more research done and money spent on new discoveries for a hopeful cure. Medications have been improved and patients are living longer lives. So I kept this story to myself all these years for you might be labeled that you were contagious or you suffered with it too.

I live with a rare thyroid cancer and I have an unknown prognosis. I started writing my cancer journey then decided to share my brother's story with you first. The following story is a journal of his illness that I wrote to de-stress and to cope with losing my precious brother. It takes you into the true last days of a patient living and dying of A.I.D.S. (Acquired Immune Disease Syndrome).

Hospital Experience of a Person with AIDS-when so little was known about this disease.

AUGUST 1986

Nicholas was admitted in the hospital Sunday, August 17,1986 at about 7:30 p.m. We took him there about 1:30. He was complaining of chest pain and fever. After blood tests, x-rays, and temperature were taken, he was admitted to the 12th floor. Dr. Klesmer was one of the doctors who examined him in the emergency room. Dr. Curti is one of his current doctors.

Monday, August 18th, the diagnosis was pneumonia-both lungs were filled with fluids. He was breathing heavy and his temperature fluctuated from 103 to 99 degrees-high/low/high. He was given an oxygen mask, which he controlled himself., a mask, not nose plugs.

Several doctors examined him daily. Blood tests and temperature were taken consistently. Heart rate and respiratory rate were monitored.

Andrea (his girlfriend) was by his bedside every moment she could spare. She brought him candy and helium balloons with cute sayings. He received get-well cards from people at work. Everyone sent his or her regards and wishes for his speedy recovery.

A priest visited and spoke with Nick and Andrea. Nick has a nutritionist who advises him about his caloric intake. He can eat as much as he wants. He drank fruit punches, liquids and shakes (240 calories each drink). We visited him from 6:20-8:20

He was very weak, pale and frail. I called mom and told her about Nick. She said she would pray for him.

Tuesday, August 19th, I was off from work. My sister-in-law, Dianne and I visited Nickey from 1:45 to 4:30 p.m. Andrea stayed all day.

We spoke to Dr. Curti. Nickey's heart and liver seemed to be okay. They were still investigating what organ pneumonia originated in. Several blood tests and x-rays were taken.

There was not enough oxygen was going through his blood. He had difficulty breathing, He was pale, tired loss of appetite and dizzy. The mask had to be kept on at all times. They were considering putting him in Intensive Care. He needed nursing care. He was scheduled for a bronchial scope tomorrow. The procedure removes a piece of tissue from the lung and is examined under a microscope.

We visited all day but Nickey requested we did not come back at night because he was tired and needed the rest. A beautiful plant was sent from his job.. It was tall with yellow flowers and a blue bow.

I called long lost Uncle Pete, who was Nickey's father's brother. He sent his love to Nickey and he was shocked to hear Nick was so sick. Uncle Pete called the family.

Surprisingly, Nick received a call from Aunt Gracie. She was so sorry to hear Nickey was in the hospital. We were hoping Aunt Marge would call. They said they may visit on Sunday but they never did. I was extremely exhausted and worried.

Wednesday, August 20th, the bronchial scope was scheduled. He was heavily sedated and awake for the test. Andrea and I visited Nickey. He was weak, groggy and breathing heavy. They did blood work and x-rays. About 12:45,they gave Nick two injections (one in the arm and one in the rear) and prepared him for the bronchoscope test.

He was sent down at 1:30. He was frightened and we were frightened for him. He was not allowed to eat anything last night or all day. He pleaded for water but his throat had to be dry for the test. (I did not quite understand why). He was told the test would be painful and uncomfortable and it was painful and uncomfortable, he said.

They had to put a tube down his throat and I believe through his nose to scope the lung and remove a piece of tissue to be diagnosed under a microscope. It felt like forever before they wheeled him back up to his room. He slept and awoke very groggy about 4:30p.m. He said the test was awful. He said he had to be awake for it. Then, they took more blood work and chest x-rays. Also, before the test, he was spitting up blood. He could not eat until about 2 hours after the test and even still the food were liquids because sometimes people react by vomiting. He had 103 fever.

Our dear friend, Jean C. (coincidentally, same birthday as my mother, February 19,1926) came to visit. She brought Nickey a stuffed animal dog. He named it Ralph. She also brought cookies, which he enjoyed with Jean.

He looked a little better. He was craving for a corned beef sandwich. We said, tomorrow we would bring him one. Funny thing is, we hadn't had corned beef in about 9 months and when I went shopping I had a craving for it and it was sitting in the fridge waiting to be cooked. I did a lot of shopping last week. I bought fruit, cookies, cereal, meat, etc., mainly for Nickey and he was not even home to enjoy all the good food. I thought maybe we could build him up by all the good food. Who knew he would end up in the hospital for so long?

I called mom and eased her mind. Dianne and Billy called. Our best friend, Rosanne returned our call about 11p.m. She sent her love to Nickey. I took an emergency personal day. I was exhausted and in pretty bad shape during the day.

Thursday, August 21, I went to work as tired as I was. Everyone asked about Nick. He was very well liked and even loved by many of his associates. There was so much genuine concern. Tears were in people's eyes; They said if there was anything they can do, to please call on them for help. It was so beautiful and heartwarming. Like one big happy family and one of our angels were missing and very sick in the hospital. Harriett T. started a collection to help pay for Nick's hospital bill. Everyone wanted to buy him gifts but Harriett said the money would be more useful and it would take away the worry from Nicholas when he was discharged from the hospital. It was so sweet of Harriett and everyone. I appreciated all they were doing. It helped make the situation easier. We had so much moral support.

Nickey was a lucky guy to be loved and cared for by so many people. Also, the power of prayer helped immensely and everyone prayed for his speedy recovery. I prayed to Saint Jude and God.

Nick called this morning and said, "Hurry up-visiting hours are almost over. Why aren't you here yet?" I said I had to work and I would see him later that night. Then, Nick called me at work and said." Hurry up-they are not going to let you in. Visiting hours are over soon." Then, I realized he did not know what time it was. He thought it was nighttime. He must have slept-it was only morning. He said he was hungry. He wanted mashed potatoes and a steak. Andrea spent all day with him again.. She brought him a corned beef sandwich and he ate it plus the hospital lunch and chocolate candy. His appetite was improving, Thank God!

A priest visited Nick from the church. He offered Holy Communion and confirmation. Nick refused but accepted prayer and conversation. Nick looked better. His temperature was 101 and he was able to sit up. He managed to go to the bathroom with his best friend,

Bill D.'s help. Bill, Karen, Ken S. visited. They gave him cards and a headphone radio…. what a thoughtful gift.

Nick talked a little but not much of a sense of humor. And the intravenous bothered him so the nurse removed it. They put it in the other arm later. He still wore the oxygen mask but was breathing better. I felt a little better. But we were not over the critical period yet. There was a glimmer of hope. Thank you, God….

Rich and I bought cantaloupe, kiwis and peaches for Nick. He ate half a kiwi. He loves them. Rich introduced him to them last year. Nick just loved the flavor. When we left the hospital. He looked like he was dozing off. I tried seeing the doctor but he was not available. Tomorrow we would hear the bronchoscope results. I needed some sleep. I had to get up early for work.

Vinnie S. gave Nick $50 to help with the hospital bill. Elaine gave $20 to help pay for the television in his room.

Everyone contributed money. It was so very thoughtful of everyone. I bought a big Thank you card and hung it on the bulletin board at work. The managers were very concerned and supportive. Bill T and Dominick P., (Nickey's bosses) were real concerned.

The managers, Terry F.(Personnel Manager), Greg M., JimS., Bob F.(Operations Manager,) RickT. (Operations Manager),Gil N.,Larry F. and all the managers ask for Nick and say they are praying for him Ben C. (my wedding photographer) always showed concern and gave emotional support. Delores B. loved Nickey and always asked for him. Doris B. drove Nick back and forth to work, sometimes. Dolores Y. and Minnie P., Cecelia K always asked about Nick.. Barbara I ,.Mary G., Terri K., Lucy B., Brenda C., Carol H., Marie P., Marie D. Adrienne C., Antoinette D. ,Lynor V., Becky L., Thelma D., Pat K.,Ginny G., Betty F and Sales Audit team , Betty B.,,Phyllis F., Gertrude M. and so many others too numerous to mention send their love. Carolee sent her love on every card plus special ones personally.

Marie D. and Marie P. were very supportive. Marie P.and I used to travel on the bus to work. We both did not drive in those days. Before Nick got sick, he would often travel and sit with us on the bus.

We shared a lot of stories about life. Marie was a good listener, which helped me release some of my pent up emotions before facing the workday.

I always believed, you leave your troubles at home when you go to work. "Cry inside and smile at the world!"

Terri K.(Assistant Personnel Manager) was an anchor of support. She knew about my life and she knew what I was facing everyday.

Terri wrote me recently and reminded me of all the lives I've touched in a positive way. She remembers me working, going to college, and taking care of Nickey and Rich Jr., my mother and so many others. She admires my strength and she says,"Barbara, you are a survivor!'

Everyone was so concerned and so genuine. The moral support was phenomenal.

I had to stay strong to pull Nick through this crisis and keep my own life in tact at work and home. I thanked God and Saint Jude and went to sleep.

Friday, August 22, Nicholas improved with each day-got a little stronger. His temperature was 102. It still fluctuates but it was getting lower.

Andrea spent all day with Nick. He was able to wash up and shave his beard. Just by shaving, he looked better and on his way to recovery.

Nick was moved from the 12th floor to the 11th floor this afternoon., Room 1158. He was moved so he could get better care-more doctors and nurses.

He talked with a psychiatrist about his depression and unhappiness in life. He had to understand how very sick he was-a very bad viral pneumonia caused by the dreaded and little known disease A.I.D.S.-certainly nothing to fool around with.

He had extensive lung damage. He gets tired easily and will be short-winded. Thank God, he quit smoking. He started when he was 11 or 12 years old

The bronchoscope showed no cancer. There were so many names for pneumonia that they could not pinpoint which one he had. They said it was a very serious viral pneumonia. His temperature was 100.9.

Elaine visited Nick with me and he was so glad to see her. Jean C.visited and brought him a soda and a mass card.

Nick still has the oxygen mask but he was able to control it as he needed it.

We thought the crisis might be over as he was reacting very well to the medication. Bactrin and Zantac were still intravenously administered.

Dr. Curti said he would be in the hospital at least another 3 weeks., Dr. Curti said he was confident that Nick would get up and walk out of the hospital recovered from this pneumonia.

That was such good news and Dr, Curti was a super doctor. He was very honest with straight forward-no bullshit.

We told him, if he had his own practice, we would be his first patients and for my husband Rich to say that and that was confidence. He did not have a lot of belief in doctors due to other illnesses in the family.

Dr. Curti was 32 years old-premature gray newly married. He said his wife never sees him. He said he smokes.... I said, "Shame/shame.... A doctor who smokes"....

He said a lot of my physical ailments were probably stress-related. He was concerned about my I.T. P.(idiothrombocytopenia purpura) count. I was having trouble with my platelets but I managed to get it under control through good nutrition and supplements.

Nick was tested for Cancer but the bronchoscope showed no cancer... that was good news. Dorothy T.gave Nick $10 and visited him at the hospital.

Everyone is being so very supportive. I don't know how to thank all these wonderful people

Please accept my heartfelt apology if I do not mention your name in this story. You were all loved and appreciated .

All my associates and friends helped me more than you know to get us through this tragic illness. Thank you everyone. Special thanks today to Carolee Jean, Elaine and Dorothy.

And one big thank you card for the entire store, Roosevelt Field Garden City, L.I.

Greg M. now (Regional Manager) always asked how I was holding up. He always said," hang in there"…. so sweet. Jim S. (now store manager) always asked about Nick. Mr. S. (then store manager) was always very concerned and so was Mr. F. (then operations manager) and Gil N.(General Manager)

Nick was getting better. I was thinking more positive. He had to gain weight before he was released.

Andrea's parents wanted us to come for lunch and discuss how Nick was doing.

My mother was terribly upset. Her son was very ill in the hospital and now her 3rd husband was put on the critical list, removed from all life support. They said any day now, he would die.

This was the hardest decision I ever had to make, signing the paper to remove him from all life support so he would not suffer anymore.

Saturday, August23, I called Nick. He was given tranquilizers to relax and calm him down. He was feeling very depressed. Andrea visited him all day. I had to work so I never got to the hospital.

Sunday, August 24, Andrea visited Nick. Rich and I brought him orange juice, cookies, peaches and plums. He was tired and depressed. His friends, Paul M. Bill D., Karen and Kevin visited him.

Monday August25, Andrea visited Nick. They both went to a group session and it was good therapy for them.

Our mother's third husband died

I received bad news at work about 3:00 in the afternoon. My mother's 3rd husband, Mike K. died of liver cancer. Rich and I had to drive to NYC to see mom and help her with the funeral arrangements. My mother's husband had no family that responded to his death. I called a few family members and did not want to help me. So here with all that's going on in our lives, Rich and I had to make funeral arrangements and bury her husband. She was only married to him about 2 years. He was legally blind and they lived in a building, called Associate of the Blind.

The only good thing that came out of her 3rd marriage was she ended up with security. She inherited the apt. Which was subsidized by the state. She lives in a 1-bedroom apt., on the 10th floor and she is safe and secure. Her husband had no money or possessions to leave her but the apartment was a Godsend.

My mother was incapable of making the funeral arrangements. I was so torn and stressed. I wanted to be with Nickey. We were not able to see Nick to tell him what happened. The doctors advised us not to tell Nick any bad news. He did not understand why I was not home when he called. Nick was tranquilized.

Tuesday August 26, Nick called several times and asked me to come visit him. He didn't realize what I was going through. I had been on the phone all day with the social worker, funeral director, Social Security, VA, mom, the bank, etc. After making all the calls, I got dressed and took a taxi to the hospital. I did not drive in those days so I walked, rode buses, caught a ride or took a taxi, which added to my stressful life. I visited with Nick. He was all doped up, feeling tired and depressed. His temperature climbed to 103.6-quite high. It had been fluctuating from 99 to 103. The doctors requested blood tests in both arms to check for bacteria. Dr. Curti showed concern about Nick's depression. I met several nurses and aides-

Wilma- very sweet-religious and philosophical

Jackie- sweet but tough-she did not stand for any nonsense

Carol- head nurse- she was good. She made Nick sit up for ½ hour in the chair instead of lying in the bed all day.

Eartha-nice-nurses aide.

And, I met Janice Driscoll, the social worker. She seemed genuinely concerned about her patients. I liked her. Supposedly a psychologist tried talking to Nick but he did not want to talk.

It was a dark and dreary day. I saw the light; the light was brighter than sunshine. I was at my wits end, deeply depressed and under so much stress. I turned on channel 9 about 7:00a.m. to the 700 Club. It is a prayer show.

At that moment my life was being broadcasted, but it wasn't I who was there. It was a person with very similar thoughts, feelings and emotions.

At first, I thought I was dreaming but I woke up to reality. I cried out to God to help me overcome the pain and suffering, depression and despair.

Then,, I felt alone until I bowed my head and began to pray.

I felt a blanket slowly covering my pain and I felt filled with the Holy Spirit.

AUGUST TO SEPTEMBER 1986

Wednesday August 27th to Sept. 10th, Nick improved with each day. He was eating a little better. His temperature continued to heighten and drop up until the last week when he was finally released from the hospital. Nick had an allergic reaction to the bactrin as well as the penicillin. This is one of the reasons for his long stay in the hospital. He was getting worse instead f better. Finally, they put him on another medication and it worked. His temperature broke and stayed normal. His breathing was easier and he was eating. Before he was discharged, they removed the iv. and the oxygen for a few days to see how he functioned without it. Andrea brought Nick home.

I didn't even know he was home until late that night., upon my return home from a business dinner for

LucyB. It was a farewell party. It was hard to believe she quit her job after 11 years of devoted work.

Nick has been home for almost a week and he was on his way to recovery from the pneumonia. He was eating better and drank his shakes with every meal he took sleeping pills to ensure proper rest and other medications.

Thank God he survived. Prayer is very powerful and pray is what we did day and night. We had a long road ahead but we were on our way to a recovery.

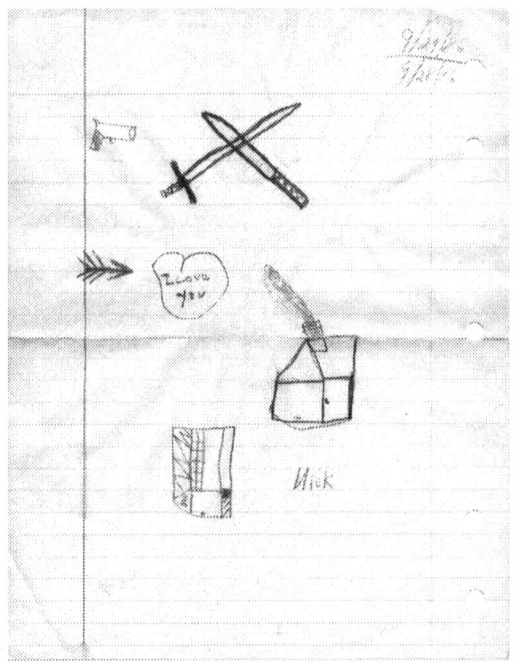

This meaningful drawing was found in Nickey's room by Barbara shortly after being discharged from the hospital. To which left many thoughts portrayed. Could this mean his life?

October 1986

Wednesday, October 15th, Nick went for an examination. He showed signs of anemia and lost weight. He was thin and drawn,126 lbs. His blood gases were normal but he had shortness of breath. He had a kidney infection ,a prostrate infection, pain in his back and difficulty urinating. Dr. Pellegrini and Dr.. Agins scheduled nick for another appt. Tuesday October 21 and 22nd,Nick had chest x-rays and renal ultrasound.

Nick was very tired and weak and had a loss of appetite,pains in his stomach and back spoke with Dr. Pellegrini. The results showed abnormalities in the blood, dysfunctions in the liver. My tooth broke off and I had to rush to the dentist for a dental emergency. I called mom. She was still having complications with her financial concerns. She needed our help. She said she is trying to cut back on her drinking and she takes long walks.

Monday, October 27th, Nick was injected with fluid for a Gallian scan at 8a.m.

Tuesday, October 28th, more x-rays were taken.

Wednesday October 29th, X-rays of stomach and lungs were taken. Dr. Pellegrini called me at work and said Nick's liver enzymes worsened. The stomach x-ray showed a possible tumor. Nick had to be admitted again.

Thursday, October 30th, Nick felt dizzy and had pains in his stomach. He went to the emergency room at 8a.m. and was admitted.

November 1986

Wednesday November 5th, So far Nick has been in the hospital almost a week. He was in pain in his stomach and back. He was very tired and weak. His liver was swollen and his liver enzymes were very high. Sunday, he had a fever,101.5. he took sleeping pills to sleep. His appetite was drastically reduced. He was receiving water and sugar intravenously. A bone marrow test was recommended. Nick refused. A catscan was scheduled for Monday. Bloodtests everyday, temperature and urine samples daily. He was scheduled for another bronchoscope but it was canceled. The pneumonia was gone. Nick was irritable,frightened and very sick.

Thursday, November 6th, Nick was weak. They gave him vitamin K to build his bloodcells back up. He was scheduled for a bone marrow test on Friday.

Friday, November 7th, I visited Nick in the morning. There was a birthday party for Larry ,one of the patients. Nick looked jaundice and very weak. He was angry and nasty. The bone marrow test was very painful.

Discharged From The Hospital

He was discharged Friday night and took a cab home. Dr. Pellegrini said the platelet count was low, but not dangerously low. His red blood count was stable but low. His white blood count was low. His liver seemed to be improving. He was prescribed benadryl ,bactrin, myclex and lozenges.

Saturday and Sunday, Nick stayed in bed. He drank water, tea and milk. He hardly ate anything. He had pain in his stomach and back.

Monday, November 10th, I woke up with a headache and nausea. I stayed home with Nick. He looked a little better. He took a shower and had hot tea, buttered roll, vitamins and medicine. His stomach was bloated. He suffered with back and stomach pain. He could hardly walk without falling. His eyes were bloodshot and yellow. Doctors were unavailable to give us results of recent medical tests.

Tuesday, November 11th, Nick's condition worsened. He was so weak and had no appetite. His equilibrium was off. He fell over the endtable in the bedroom. He had pains in his stomach.

Wednesday, November 12th, Nick looked bad. He was very jaundice and could hardly walk. He fell over everything.... He was so dizzy. He had pain in his legs and stomach and no appetite.

Thursday, November 13th, Nick was still falling. He could not walk. He was off balance. He had a nosebleed. His stomach was bloated and very jaundice. Dr. Lebowitz said if the situation is that bad to bring him into the emergency room. Nick refused to go. Nick requested frosted flakes cereal, peaches and chocolate chip cookies. He also wanted ice-cream, 7-up and Pepsi.

Friday, November 14th, Nick wanted ice-cream and chocolate chip cookies. He was off balance,had pains in his stomach nose bleed and rectal bleeding. He took a bath ,ate his favorite platanos,drank 7-up,pepsi,tea. His stomach was bloated and he had difficulty walking. He held onto the walls to go to the bathroom. He was frightened. He still refused to go to the hospital. He said he feels safe with me.

Saturday. November 15th, 4a.m., Nick had rectal bleeding and pains in his stomach. He took a bath and had frosted flakes cereal, spilling some on the floor, accidentally.

He had coffee and orange juice and said he would go to the hospital tomorrow. The store collected money and we bought food plaid maroon pajamas, maroon robe and maroon slippers so Nick could stay comfortable and warm. I was so tired. I never sleep anymore, between work and college it has been so difficult.

Saturday, November 15, Nick was still in pain and was bleeding. He promised he would go to the hospital. He looked real bad and could hardly walk. Nick called me at work and said there was a pool of blood all over the chair. I tried calling an ambulance and the hospital said to call 911. I called and got a busy signal. I was desperate. I didn't want to call my sister-in-law Dianne because her father just died and they were having the funeral. I called a family friend, Terri M.. Terri went to my house and talked Nick into going to the emergency room ,with great resistance. She helped him get dressed and rushed him over.

NICK WAS READMITTED IN THE HOSPITAL

From what I understand, they took him right in. He was still bleeding from the rectum. They did a proctoscope and admitted him to ICU He needed blood transfusions because he lost a lot of blood. He was on the second floor in unit 4.

Bill and Dianne picked me up from work and I stayed with them for the weekend. Bill talked to a consultant in I..C. U. Rich was hunting for the weekend.

NICK WAS IN CRITICAL CONDITION

Sunday, November 16th, Nick was in critical condition. He was in ICU., had blood transfusions,I.V. feedings. His heart was monitored and it was strong. He had mental confusion. He just mumbled. It was so sad. We visited twice that day. Nick was in very bad shape.

Monday, November 17th, I visited about 2:00. Spoke with Dr. Lambert who I was not thrilled about. He walked away from me in the middle of the conversation. I guess I asked him questions he could not answer. I asked to speak to his superior, Dr. Foto. He was very nice and showed a little compassion. I called Dr. Pellegrini and he was glad I did. He said he could not believe the turnabout of events. He said it was pancreatic cancer,fluids were building up in Nick's stomach and his liver is shot.The heart was going strong. I had to consent to two tests immediately spinal tap and a lumbar to check the stomach fluids. It might be affecting the brain as Nick had mental confusion and hallucinations.   I visited Nick about 7p.m.. He was given more blood transfusions,clear fluids and Demerol for the pain. His liver was not functioning and the enzymes were very high. Andrea visited him in the afternoon. She was very upset to see in this condition as we all were.

Darrin was assigned as a caretaker to Nick. He was wonderful. Thank God for Darrin. He was always so helpful ,compassionate, honest and firm. He really took good care of Nick. He cleaned his room ;emptied his drawers and put all the clothes back neatly folded. He did his laundry and he made Nick platanos which Nick barely touched. Darrin gave a lot of T. L.C. which Nick needed.

Barbara:

Nick really needs to be in the hospital. He can not take care of himself. I tried to convince him of this - but he did not wish to listen.

His room was horrible - I did his laundry and cleaned his room, closet and drawers.

He seemed to be hungry - I made him pancakes for lunch - He did not really touch it, however,

I arrived about 10:00 and left about 3:00 p.m.

Good luck with Nick - call if you need anything - and try to get him to go back to the hospital.

Darren

God Bless Nick and I wish he didn't have to suffer anymore. I asked, Why is God making him suffer so much? He was such a good person...an angel in disguise. Part of me said to take him to heaven and part of me said I could not let go. I called our sister Lana. She is quite upset and knows how bad I felt about all this. My stomach was always in a knot and I was hardly ever able to sleep. When I did try, I cried myself to sleep.

Tuesday, November 18th, Richie Jrs 15th birthday. I woke him up and got him off to school. Rich sr. Is still sleeping. I called our jobs. We could not make it in to work. Maybe after the test results, maybe if we find another glimmer of hope.We are scared. I pray God does not let him suffer anymore. Maybe his father Mike is calling him home. Or maybe our dear friend Rommie in heaven does not want us to shed anymore tears. Maybe Nick is being punished for the past. We told my mother and she took it really bad.,especially a week before Thanksgiving. Oh, my God, we prayed. I just called Sister Theresa and she prayed for Nick that he would not suffer anymore. She prayed for God to give me the strength to endure. I called Andrea and she was very upset. Andrea and I went to the hospital. Nick was in critical condition. I spoke with Janice Driscoll, social worker. She said she did not know how I was handling all this standing up. She said it was ego strength that I have.

Nick as out of I.C. U. and back on the 11th floor. Dr. Dwarte was the covering doctor. He was informative and nice. Spoke with dr. Foto. He said the liver was not functioning and the enzymes were very high, confirming pancreatic cancer.

Wednesday, November 19th to November 26th. Nick was intravenously fed. A waterbed was ordered for him. He suffered a lot of mental confusion. And was in a lot of pain. He was not allowed to eat. His mouth broke

out, he had sores, dehydrated and very thin. More or
less he was confined to bed. Bill D. visited often. Nick
says he was his best friend. He sat with Nick for an
hour or more at a time. Paul M. visited when he could.
Steve H. visited .Nick had a craving for lifesavers so we
bought him packs of them-all flavors. We should have
bought stock in the company. Darrin visited when he
could. He always was nice and cared for Nick. Bill and
Dianne called all the time. Terri called. Chris was very
concerned. Mom was so upset. She said," my only son,
why"? Lana's upset.

JENNIFER SENT UNCLE NICKEY A LETTER AND HER CHERISHED ROSARY BEADS

My niece, Jenny is very upset. She wrote her Uncle Nick a letter and sent her cherished rosary beads to him. She said she loved her uncle Nickey and did not want him to die. But, if he did die, she wanted him to wear these rosary beads around his neck forever.

My nephew Dennis had an epileptic seizure when he found out. There's a lot of tension all around. We are so tired.

Nick looked better the other night but the doctor said his liver enzymes were climbing everyday. 300 should be 30-40. He had a lot of mental confusion.

Dr. Simms is the new doctor on the case. He seems to be very concerned and very caring. He was always there when I called.

Nick had a build up of fluids again and his stomach was protruding. They might drain the fluids.

RICH JR WAS SUSPENDED FROM SCHOOL

Wednesday, November 26th, Rich Jr. Was suspended from school. He was caught smoking. He says he smoked a pack a day. Who knew? We were so wrapped up in working and nick being so sick, we neglected our son. I never thought he would smoke. He always hated his father smoking. I knew he would drink but never thought he would smoke. We had to meet with the assistant principal. She was very nice. She said Rich Jr. was a nice boy and he growing up well but we had to nip it in the bud now, His grades were poor this quarter. He even went down in his favorite subject, Science and failed Gym. We signed him back in school and hoped this was the last of it. She was very understanding as we explained our family trauma with Nick.

We were all so exhausted. I looked terrible. I lost a lot of weight. I had breakfast and took vitamins. Swallowed a tranquilizer to get through the day. I had another long day ahead of me.

I called Nick. He just got back from a sonogram. He was still not able to eat. He drank lactose (milk sugar) which gives him violent diarrhea. We could only hope it helped to flush out his system. This is horrible. I feel so bad for Nick.

A long time friend, Betty L. visited on Monday. She is the sweetest lady you want to meet. She is gentle and kind and an angel in disguise. She brought Nick a teddy bear. He was afraid someone would take it so he asked me to take it home for him and keep it safe.

Nick was in and out of consciousness. I stayed with him for a few hours. Nick knew I was there. He opened his eyes as soon as he heard my voice. I loved Nick so very much and I also know he loved me. Because he responded to me and my voice always. He had a little fighting spirit. I promised I would bring his stuffed animal dog I bought him the first Christmas he was with us.

I went to work late on Wednesday. Greg M.spoke with me that evening. He was so warm, kind and supportive. He said he was surprised I had been working all this time under these conditions. Nick had visitors, Bill D., Paul and Steve.

What Was There to be Thankful For?

Thursday, November 27th was Thanksgiving. What was there to be thankful about? Nick was in the hospital dying. We woke up very early. It was a beautiful clear sunny day. To me it was a picture of heaven-the birds were flying in the sky and everything was so peaceful. It was the calm before the storm, much like a thief in the night going to the angel in the light. My interpretation being A.I.D.S was the thief in the night taking my brothers life but he would meet an angel in the light of heaven. I knew it was inevitable. I cried the entire day.

Rich B. And I Prayed Together At The Hospital

Our good friend, Richard Branker and I visited Nick at about 11:20 in the morning. Rich said it was Thanksgiving and he needed to pray with Nick. Nick was sleeping peacefully. He did wake up for water. I gave him a sip of water and he seemed to be grateful.

Nick complained of a little abdominal pain in the morning and the doctor gave him something for it. His temperature was normal for a change but his blood pressure was low. WE only stayed a little while but I think he felt our presence.

Nickey Wanted To Come Home

Rich and I did laundry and afterwards, we visited Nick. He was sleeping peacefully. He did wake up for soda and Rich ran to get him a soda. He drank a can of Gingerale. And, he said he wanted to go home. The doctor said he could leave with us, Nick said. He said to Rich., "Ah come on"! He wanted to come home and die where he knew family and love and security. We felt so terrible. Rich was besides himself. Rich felt so cheated. We took Nick out of a negative environment and now A.I.D.S. is stealing him away from us. Then, Nick asked for more soda-Rich bought him 2 more cans of Gingerale. And he seemed to open his eyes to a Smurf cartoon. He said Goodbye to Michael, his friend, a patient in the next bed, He must have believed he was coming home with us. I cried all day. I felt like I was losing nick faster and faster. He was slipping away. The doctor said he was slipping away. The doctor said he was in very bad condition and there was nothing they could do medically to help him. What a prognosis.

I did not even know what I shoveled in my mouth for dinner at Bill and Dianne's house. They put a plate in front of me and I went through the motions. I had 2 vodkas and we went to bed early. I just wanted the world to go away. The phone rang and rang and I did not answer it. The doorbell rang and I did not answer it.

Friday, November 28th, I woke up early and called the hospital. The nurse, Barbara Doran told me I'd feel very bad if something happened and I didn't take the time off work and be there with Nick. She said pray on it but Nick was in very bad condition. His liver failed, he had mental confusion, unable to talk or swallow. Here it was the busiest day in Retailing and my brother was dying. I was numb.

Helen K. picked me up and I decided to go to work but I also decided to leave by noon. Barbara I.and I sat down and had something to drink. She was very concerned about me as everyone was. I told her I had to leave. I was very matter a fact about it. I let my boss Mr. Florence know as soon as he walked in the cafeteria. He said okay and he understood. Thank God,I had the sense to leave early from work. I left about 12:15 with Elaine. She was leaving early and offered me a ride to the hospital.

Before we went to the hospital. Elaine and I stopped at Friendly's for lunch. We hadn't really talked in quite awhile since we were both always on the run and going in different directions. Of course, we fought over who would pay the bill and she won. She treated me to lunch. It came to $9.99-how weird-we thought it was kind of strange.

Elaine and I Visited Nickey at The Hospital

It was another beautiful day . Elaine and I went to the hospital and the doctors said he was very critical. He probably wouldn't last the weekend. His liver stopped functioning and it was so small besides. They couldn't believe how fast nick was deteriorating. I believe it was the power of prayer. God, please release Nick from his suffering and take him home with you. He did make peace with God several times. And, I believe our prayers were answered.

The nurse, Barbara Doran wouldn't let us walk in alone. She came with us and told me to pay strict attention to his coloring. Nick actually looked good. He looked like he had an all around tan. He looked like he came back from a cruise to Jamaica or the Bahamas or one of those exotic Islands. As soon as he heard our voices, he was aroused. He looked so peaceful lying there. He really did not look like he was in any pain.

Elaine and I cried so much in each others arms. We cried for him and we cried for all the good times we had together. Elaine loved Nick and nick loved Elaine. We used to go for a drink after work or dancing or to dinner or to her house or our house. We had so many memories. Nick was not gone yet but it felt like it. Elaine held his hand and rubbed it and said, Nick you can sit in the front seat and you can listen to the radio and we are going for that beer now. And God is my witness-Nick sat up in the bed and made a motion. He tried so hard to talk, to say something. All he could do was purse his lips as if to give a kiss and who knew that was the goodbye kiss-maybe deep down inside we really did know.

Nick was so very special and he was slipping away from us. But I believe he recognized us and he knew we were there for him. Oh god, I do believe it!

Elaine and I stayed for several hours and she was glad we did. We left, drove to my house ,talked ,looked over dream and psychic predictions, talked to Rich and Elaine was on her way home. She 's such a good friend.

Rich got ready for his hunting trip. He reluctantly went hunting. He felt it like I felt it-the calm before the storm. He called the airlines and prepared a flight to fly home just in case anything happened. Nick was going this time and there was no turning back. The doctors said there was nothing they could do medically. The liver had to take its natural course, either get worse or better and the likelihood was to get worse and Nick was getting worse day by day. Rich said he would fly home within a few hours and he didn't want me to do anything until he arrived home if anything were to happen.

I was bound and determined to visit Nick, no matter what-if I had to walk, run, take a cab or whatever. I had to be with him in his final hours.

Dianne offered to come with me. Thank God we went. We stayed for about 3 hours. Everyone was there by his bedside. Bill D.(his best friend),Karen, Jean C.,(god love her), Debbie S., Dianne and I.

The Goodbye Kiss

We rallied around his bedside and it was the last time. When Karen kissed him on the forehead, I knew it was the kiss goodbye. It was final. I felt it in my bones. I felt it in my heart. I believe somehow Nick knew we were there. He made motions and he tried so hard to speak. He was too weak. He probably wanted to say Goodbye-thank you. I love you.

Dr. Simmons stayed hours beyond the call of duty. He did not want to leave Nick's bedside. He was hoping he would turn around-that some miracle would happen-that he would see a glimmer of hope-a touch of improvement but things just got worse. Nick's blood pressure was very low and he was breathing shallow. We knew this was it.

Final...Goodbye Nick. Goodbye and we loved you so very much. I didn't want to leave. I wanted to be there until the last moment. I wanted him to know that I loved and cared for him from when he was born to his young death. I wanted him to know he wasn't alone in the world. He was my life. He made everything worthwhile. I never let him grow up until maybe this past year when I thought he was ready. To me he was my child and I feel such a loss. We finally got him to the point of soaring on his own. He was just about ready to leave and marry Andrea and have a life of his own without me. And Rich always being there. So very unfair-He was a little boy in a mans body and maybe that's the way I wanted him to stay. It gave me a purpose. I watched him grow, change, develop and I was so proud of him. He was very proud of himself. He was proud of his family life. He was proud of his job, his friends, his girlfriend, Andrea, his freedom, his independence. He was proud of his room. He was proud of his clothes. He was proud of his music equipment that he paid for himself.

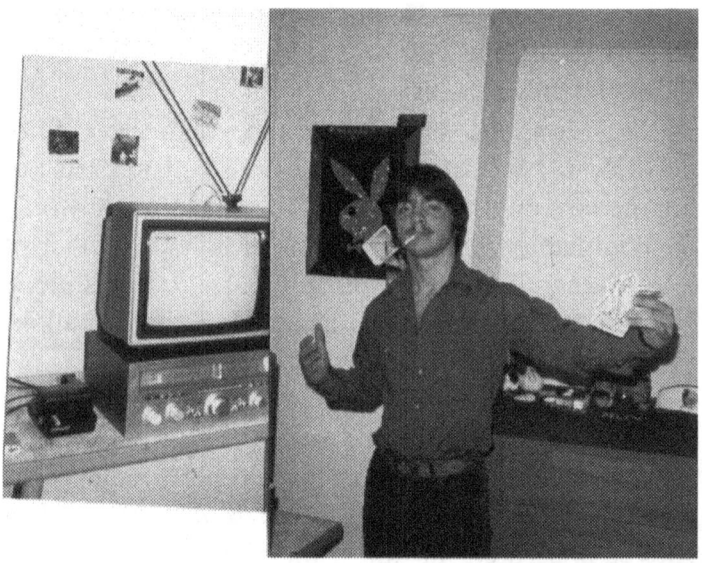

He died in style. Oh God, I love him so…. I still have not accepted it. I still think he is in the hospital and he's being well taken care of. God help me when it hits me. I 'm like a robot right now. I kept myself very busy. I have tears in my eyes right now as I am writing this.

The Dreaded Phone Call-
Nickey Died-
November 29, 1986.

When the phone rang Saturday morning, I didn't want to know but I knew. Dr. DiSalvo(covering doctor) said, "Barbara I am sorry to inform you but your brother expired this morning at 3:15a.m" Thank God I decided to stay at Diannes with her and Theresa and Wheat and Gina. I really wanted to be by myself for the weekend but Dianne insisted and I was to weak to resist. I really haven't had much sleep since that phone call. I was exhausted. My eyes hurt so much. They were burning. We called Rich upstate and he flew home within a few hours. He looked like hell and so did I but we knew what had to be done. It was over and nick lived 4 years of quality. He always said he would live fast and die young-22 years old-so very unfair. He was just starting his life.

Planning The Funeral

Anyway that set the chain of events to come. By noon, Rich and I had the funeral arrangements started. We decided to have a one-day service (wake) Monday. We figured by Saturday we would be able to contact everyone and contact everyone is what we did. The phone never stopped ringing and our phone bill was over $200. We called New Jersey, Florida and New York City, Upstate NY, Breezy Point, Wantagh, Garden City, etc.

Everyone is coming Monday to Thomas D. Dalton Funeral Home. The mass was held on Tuesday at 9:45a.m. St. Bernard's Church., Levittown, L.I.

And, we had him cremated afterwards. Rich had discussed cremation with Nick many times. He wanted it to be done rather than be buried in the ground. Rich will take his ashes and spread them over the ocean or a mountain one day where he will be peaceful. He's in our hearts and always will be.

I am amazed at how many lives Nick has touched in such a loving and positive way and in such a short lifespan. I could probably make a movie of his life as he always wanted to be an actor and he would have been a good one.

Donna, one of Nick's girlfriends always said, Nick reminded her of the actor, James Dean. She said it was his body language and his expressions.

I wanted to title this book, LIVE FAST, DIE YOUNG but somebody wrote a book about James Dean, using this title in 1997. He was handsome, smart and personable. He was energetic.

My Aunt Shirley remembers visiting Nickey in our South Bronx apartment and how he showed her he could do tumblesaultsand double tumblesaults as a young child, which showed he had gymnastic abilities. His favorite color was blue. Our mother used to say," Blue, Blue, God loves you.', He loved chocolate and strawberry ice-cream.

Rich and I are hurting and so is Rich Jr.The hurt never goes away. I was very surprised but Rich Jr wanted to move into Nickeys room. I guess he wanted to be closer to him. He said he wanted to talk about him at the mass and the wake. How very special. Rich gave me a big kiss and hug and said how sorry he was to hear about Nick.

Nickey's Funeral

If a funeral could be beautiful-Nick's was beautiful. We had the wake for one day Monday afternoon and evening-open casket. He looked very good.

People filled the room every minute of the day. Lee P. and her friend Helen W. drove in (each carrying their canes) from New Jersey to pay their last respects. Terry F. Personnel manager, (now store manager) let anybody from the store go when they wanted to. All the bosses came -even the store manager, Mr. S .It was wonderful. They couldn't believe how strong I was and how I was holding up. Mr. S. said,"Barbara, you have the strength of 5 men." People just didn't know what to say to me. I was so glad everyone came to the funeral.

My dear friend, Diane C. remembers Nickey's funeral and the stories I told about Nick at the funeral.

There was not a dry eye in the place. There were so many people, flowers and Mass cards.

Diane remembers Nick in 1983 having fun in her pool with Rich Jr. At her Memorial Day get-together in

Medford, L.I. And now to see him in the coffin at 22. It seems like a lifetime ago….

Joanne G. and Richard B. are very good family friends. Nick lived with us in their house in Levittown, L.I. (We rented an apartment from them, after moving from Lee and Rommie's house in Wantagh. L.I.).

JoAnne smiles every time she remembers hearing Nickey's voice, "I swear to God"…"I swear to God", after almost everything he said.

Nick was very special to JoAnne and Rich. They miss him.

Jimmy K. remembers Nickey telling him a story about taking a guys car for a ride around the block. The guy looked distressed so, Nickey said, "What's wrong?" The guy said, "I can't find my car." Nickey said, "Well, if you give me $100,I will see if I can find your car." The guy did not believe Nickey but, Nickey brought the car back and the guy gave Nickey $75 for finding his car. Nickey said to Jimmy, "See, there's all kinds of ways of making money on the streets of NYC."

Bill Kimbley said," I remember you and Rich nurturing Nickey. He was such a beautiful kid. It was so sad to see him wasting away in the hospital. He had his whole life ahead of him.' Nickey told Bill he was so happy to finally have love, security and a happy home.

Paul Kimbley (President of the Club) remembers the good times we had at the Merrick Rod and Gun Club, Seaford, L.I. Nickey joined us for the barbecues and parties. He was a good kid.

Ron K. said," Nickey was a kid who wanted to be happy and accepted. He had a hard life ,living in NYC. He loved life and he lived life." Ron went to a few nightclubs with Nick and had some good times. They dated some girls before Nick fell in love with Andrea. Through the years, Ron had some misunderstandings with Nick but, they worked it out. Ron liked Nick. They grew up in different schools of life, Nick from the big city and Ron from Long Island. Ron said," Nick and I would have been best buddies if we went to the same school or grew up in the same neighborhood. "

John Kimbley said, "Barbara when you write this book about Nickey, leave no stone unturned. His life story needs to be shared with everyone.````

Chris McClary emailed me recently : Dear Sis, "I tried to write down a few things but it only repeated what you already said about Nick. He was sweet and loving and so proud of what he was able to have in his short and hard life. You and Rich gave him the greatest gift , your love for him without judgment"

"My sorrow is that I was not able to be there for you both during the hardest parts, his passing and suffering. This left a big hole in your lives, after giving Nick so much opportunity. '

"The video of Nick was good because Nick was good. He said it all in those few minutes of film as if he knew then that his time was coming. "

"Nick passed on just when the AIDS epidemic was waving through the country. Everyone was afraid of getting AIDS. If it happened now, Nick might still be here with us. "

"You and Rich stuck it out and did all you could do, at the hardest time. You did not let go and I believe

Nick held on longer because of your love and devotion for him. Love you Sis and Rich very much. This was a brave and hard task for you to perform." Love, Sis

Bill D. (Nickey's best friend), from Long Island says every time he drives down the Wantagh Parkway, he looks over at the Levittown house and thinks of Nick. The memories come flooding back In Loving Memory... You're in Our Heart Always, Love, Billy and Karen

Bill married Karen and they are celebrating their 10-year anniversary, this year, 2004. They are parents of three sons, ages, 10,7 and 5.

Nickey's good friend, Ken S., said Nick was a very dear friend and he would miss him dearly.

I was going through mass and sympathy cards last night. I read them with tears rolling down my cheeks. Nickey and I gave our hearts to these people and they gave theirs through their love, words, good deeds and prayers.

Nickey's friends from NYC came to the funeral and gave two cards. They were Tato, Aida, Lee, Miguel and Black Boy(these were the names signed on the cards). There were two cards from Nickey's friend, Norman A.

Here are more comments from Associates, friends and acquaintances, Nickey and I both knew:

Terry F. remembers my total involvement with Nickey as if I were his mother. He remembers my courage, love and concern for my brother. Terry F. said," I always told you, Barb, family comes first and you showed that by what you did for your family; especially your mother and brother, Nickey!"

A mass card from Jim and Theresa S. that offers a prayer for everlasting peace and rest. Jim S. said", I enjoyed getting to know Nicholas and working with him."Nick and I were making achievements through the ranks.

Rick T. sent a card, saying, "Barb, I was shocked and sorrowed to hear about Nick". "May God bless you and comfort you in your grief."

Bob F. said, "Nickey was a hard worker." He remembers Nickey working in the Catalog Department with Terri G. and Gen B. and team. He also, remembers him working on the dock. Nickey was well-liked by all

Larry F. said," Nicholas was a hard worker and a good kid."

Brenda C. said, she remembers Nickey being a nervous and nice young man." He was always very helpful!"

Adrienne C. said, "Nicholas was a fantastic fellow and a joy to work with." She had many heart to heart conversations with him. He told her about his life because he trusted her. She said, "Nick, leave the past behind, look forward to the future and have a positive attitude. "

Betty B. commented, "Nicholas was a boy who went wrong but he turned out to be a nice young man. Barbara helped him get on the right track. He was honest and hardworking. Barbara gave him a beautiful farewell and a touching eulogy. "

Phyllis F. said, "Nickey came a long way from where he came from. He was well-liked and very helpful."

Bernice D. said, "Nickey was an extraordinary person. He came from the hard knocks of life and found a normal and stable life with Barbara and Richard. He made a lot of accomplishments."

Mary O. - "Nicholas was a great kid. Barbara you were a good sister to Nickey-you did all you could for him."

Lucy M. remembers picking up Nickey at the busstop, several times in the snow and ice of Winter. She would say, "Come on-Get In"! She also took him home from work a few times. She said, "Nickey was a good hearted person. God takes the good people."

Maureen M. writes, her heart reaches out in sorrow of a shared experience -the loss of a loved one in the prime of their life. She said," the love and care you gave to Nicholas has earned you the respect and admiration of all who know you. May only the happy memories of a wonderful young man remain with you."

Pauline L sent a card stating the Lord is faithful. He saved the sight of her left eye. She said, "Nick, you were always kind and respectful to me. God loves you and so do I?

Marie P and Marie D. say, "God will bless you always for your great charity and love."

Linda S. notes," Nicholas was always a special kid to me. He will always be in our prayers".

Remember the happy times and be comforted he is with you. Love, Pat K.

"I will miss Nick", Jean H.

God and all our prayers will see you through-Gen and Lori B.

You have my deepest sympathy, Love, Mae and Samantha C., Lucille R.

May God grant you all serenity and love, Joan O.

With all our thoughts and prayers, Gertrude and Joe M.

With Deepest Sympathy Rosanne and Don

In Our hearts and prayers- Love your cherished sister Barbara, Richard, Richard Jr and Mom

Dear Barbara, you were a wonderful sister to Nickey. God knows you did the best any sister could. We love you for it. May Nickey find the peace and happiness in the new world. Love from all of us.

Our mother's family came to support her and I. Shirley and Jimmy Casey, Billy and Jean Owens, Ana and Dolly and numerous cousins.

Aunt Shirley remembers Nickey being energetic and lovable.

Aunt Jeanie remembers Nickey's warm and vivacious smile.

Aunt Anne says, "I was shocked to hear about Nickey's death. It was so sad to see him die at 22. He had his whole life ahead of him." She remembers seeing him as a baby and thinking- what a good looking boy.

Aunt Dolly said, "I loved Nickey". "Nickey was a good natured kid with a great sense of humor. He was the funniest kid I ever met. It was sad to see him die so young."

Aunt Suzie met Nickey Upstate NY when he was a little boy. She remembers Nickey fixing moms hair. She commented on what a good job he did and he replied," I like my mother to always look nice."

Aunt Della always lived in Florida, but she sent a mass card. She called to express her sympathy and prayers.

She remembers visiting family in NY and meeting Nickey for the first time in the South Bronx.

Nickey was about 5 years old. She thought, what a beautiful little boy but she was shocked at his (foul) street language mouth. Nickey looked like her son Jimmy when he was a little boy.

Then she saw Nickey again, years later. He was vacationing in Florida, visiting his sister Lana and her family.

Della thought how well he turned out. He had a second chance, living with his sister Barbara, away from the memories of his traumatic childhood.

My cousin, Debbie S. (Aunt Della's daughter) sent me a card recalling how she and I sat on the beach in Florida and we talked about, how there is a reason for everything that happens to us in this life. She said, I gave Nickey a good life though it was a short time. She said, I gave him the most important thing in life… "LOVE"….

Paul Rooney Sr. said," When Nicholas was alive, I was unaware that he was HIV Positive. On several occasions, my wife Kathy and I had a few beers with Nick and we had a good time. on Long Island..

Nick told us he was originally from the city. He had a very tough childhood.

At the time, Nicholas seemed to be doing well in life. He was living with Barbara and Rich. He was working, and he had a nice girlfriend. He was thinking about going to school to get a trade. He was very protective of his family. Nick was enjoyable to be around."

Paulie Jr. (Kathy's son) said, he remembers Nickey's funeral." It wasn't Nick's fault. He had a tough life."

Mom says she loved her son. "Nickey was stern with me. Sometimes, I was afraid of him but he always tried to look out for me. I know he loved me."

My husband, Rich was wonderful. He was so strong, which is what I desperately needed. Rich Jr. was great too. It was so hard on Rich Jr. It was like losing his big brother and or his best friend.

Everyone loved Nick.

Bill and Dianne Kimbley were wonderful. They opened their house in Wantagh to us and bought all the food and everything I needed in case anyone wanted to come back to the house. We paid them back as soon as we were able to. Lenny, Bill's boss lent us $1,000 to help pay for the funeral. We paid it back.

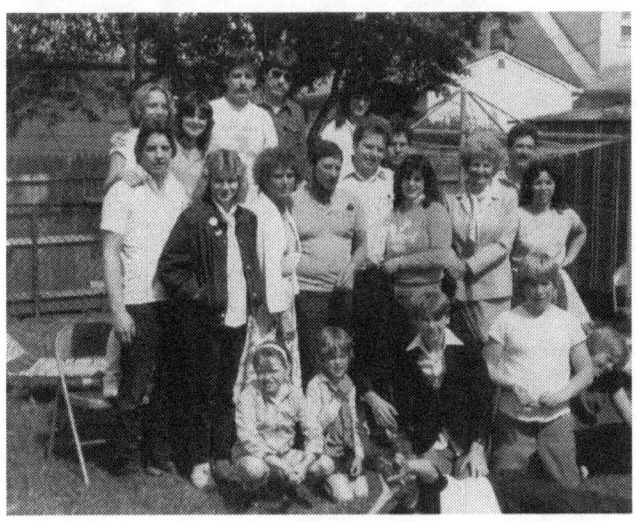

Billy, Dianne & Family

Cousin Kathy Rooney and her two children, Danielle and Paulie drove out to our apt. in Levittown, Long Island (that we rented from Joanne Greensmith and Richard Branker who became like family to us), as soon as Kathy heard and stayed with me the entire time.

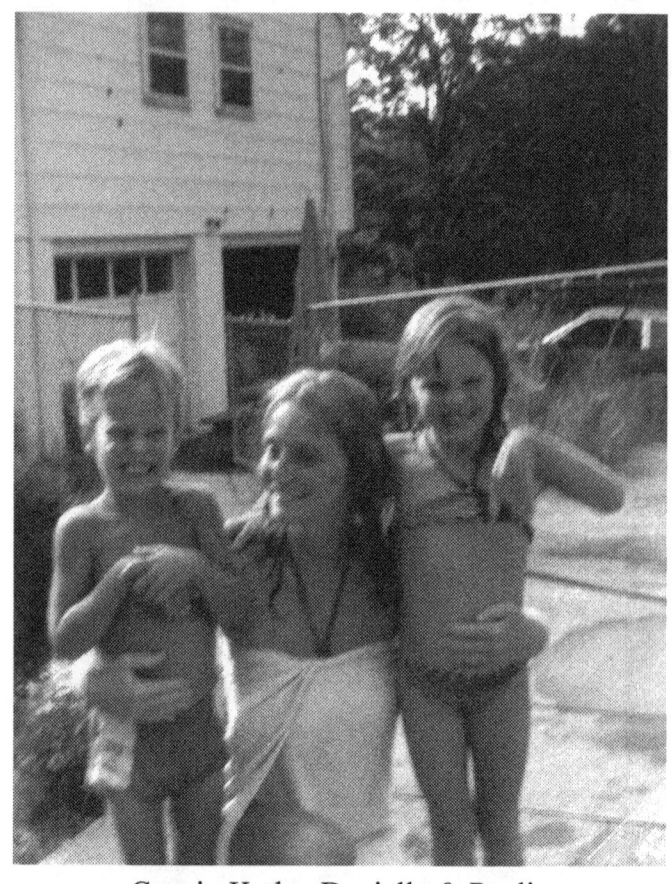

Cousin Kathy, Danielle & Paulie

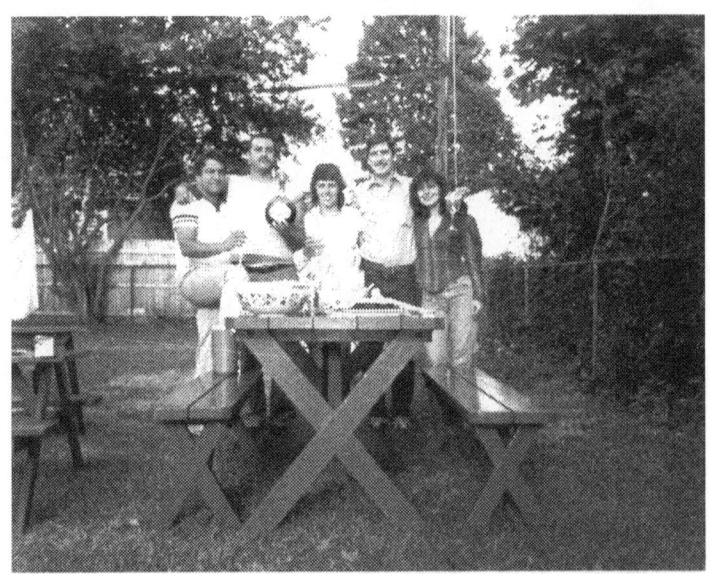

Left Richard Branker – Middle Joanne

Kathy was a big help. We took my mom shopping for clothes for the funeral. We bought her a tailored black suit with a dressy long sleeved white blouse, stockings and new black shoes. Kathy was super to me and my mother. She always has been my closest cousin and always will be. We grew up together and shared oceans of laughter and tears. She is like a sister to me. Kathy remembers when Nickey lived with her family, Shirley and Jimmy Casey in Hollis, Queens, when Nickeys parents were separated for approximately six months or more, not being the first separation, either. Shirley and Kathy were driving down 90th Avenue, going to the subway on Hillside Ave. to pick up Nickey, Barbara and Aunt Ethel, when they spotted them. Aunt Ethel, wearing her red coat(her favorite color is red)and a child in each hand. During this period, Kathy saw how attached Nickey was to his mother and how insecure he was. He always clung to his mothers hand, her skirt or pantleg, fearful of losing her. And at the time of our loss of Nickey, it just seemed so unfair how God can take a child before his own mother.

Aunt Ethel and Kathy had many conversations about Nickeys life and how he was overprotective of her. He displayed his anger and concern with the men that were involved in her life ,threatening to shoot her and them several times. Kathy further recalls, Aunt Ethel telling her of a time when Nickey's father, Mike and her were separated and Nickey was a baby,Mike climbed up the fire-escape,entering her apartment and threatening to put Nickey in the oven,if she didn't take him back. Knowing him and how one time,in a drunken angry state ,he physically picked up Barbara and held her out the 5th floor window, threatening to drop her, it was believable.

Ethel also, told a story about Nickeys compassionate side. Nickey had a cat,named Midnight that he loved. It was a big black cat with green eyes. She sat on the windowsill of Nickey's apartment ,watching everything that went on. One day, he came home and Midnight was having kittens, Nickey got a blanket and made the Midnight warm and comfortable while she delivered her kittens. He made sure the kittens and the mama cat had food and milk and were warm and safe. He nurtured them like little babies. He threatened his mom,"if anything ever happens to those kittens or Midnight,someone would pay for it"!

In the funeral home and through the mass, Kathy held Aunt Ethel's hand so she wouldn't jump in her sons coffin. She promised many times to do so. She would say,"I will jump right in...I will jump... you don't know me."' I will do it.'

All awhile in Kathy's heart and in her thoughts, she felt how rough and how very sad Nickey's life was, from beginning to end-and how far someone can come in changing his life for the better and only for it to end so abruptly.

We know Nick is in peace-safely home. I chose Father Mannion to speak at the wake. God bless him... he was wonderful. I ran up quickly and said a eulogy from a mass card that Lee gave me called SAFELY HOME. It was so very special. We loved Nicholas so very much from birth to his death.

Nick had so many friends. Flowers and mass cards filled the funeral home. He was at peace at last. It was now hard for the living.

A Heartfelt Letter To My Friends and Associates:

Wed. 12/3/86

Dearest Associates and Friends

Thank you for all the love and support you gave endlessly to Nicholas and I during this traumatic time. My message to each and everyone of you is through Nicholas's death we will find a new meaning and a new purpose for living. WE will discover that Life is too short and we must live each day to the fullest. Today is the first day of the rest of our lives. Nicholas physically died but he will live on forever in our hearts.

With Love,

Barbara

P.S. I believe Nick is safely home with God as I said to you at the wake.

Nickey's Voice and Footsteps

I heard Nick's voice one day as I walked into my empty house. He called my name-"Barbra"-'Barbra.' I saw a light shine in the kitchen window and I saw shadows and pictures in the sky during sunrise and sunset-peaceful pictures and colorful scenes. Every now and then, I hear his footsteps or his voice. I wonder what its like in heaven? It must be lovely and peaceful. He hasn't complained yet…

Isn't Life something? I go from one trauma to the next. Ironically, six months after Nickey's death, our house in Levittown, NY was burglarized.

I came home from work and I was very tired. I did not want to go out. I just wanted to stay home, eat something and go to sleep.

My husband was getting ready for his business Mans Bowling League-a night out with the guys. My sister-in-law, Dianne called and convinced me to go to dinner and to play Scrabble at her house. My husband was in a rush so I reluctantly changed my clothes to casual wear, got a ride with him and met my sister-in-law.

I was getting back on my feet again after Nickey dying and then…

We came home Tuesday, May 5,1987 to find our house robbed and ransacked. The cops say they got in through a window they pried open downstairs and then went upstairs.

The front door upstairs was busted and off the hinges, kicked in. and the bedroom door was busted and off the hinges, too. My knickknack shelf was off the wall and knickknacks were shattered on the floor. My dresser drawers were opened and the clothes were hanging out all over. The curtain was slightly open as if someone was keeping a watch-out.

Nickey's VCR, our money and jewelry were stolen. We figured this happened between 7 and 9p.m. because we left about 6:10 p.m. Joanne G. and Richard B. left about 7:00 p.m. for a short while.

What a frightening experience? The cops said they were dangerous characters. Good thing I was not home.. God works in mysterious ways. I may not have been alive to tell this story.

I found myself very paranoid and suspicious of everyone-every person, car, jogger, bicycle rider, etc. It took me over a year to get over this fright. I felt violated and fearful.

This haunts me to this day… who were they? Why did they rob me? Will they ever be caught?

Reminiscing About Our Childhood Dream

LEMONADE STORY

Years later, I was reminiscing back to our childhood. I shared my childhood dream with Nickey- one day we would fly high in the sky on a big jet to San Francisco, California.

Nickey and I SET UP A LEMONADE STAND TO MAKE MONEY SO OUR DREAM WOULD COME TRUE. Our mother, Ethel showed us how to make real good lemonade. We shopped at the fruitstand and local grocer. We bought lemons and sugar. Mom said ,"you boil the lemons in a large pot of water-when you smell the lemons you add ice and sugar-Wallah-lemonade". We looked high and low and found a large glass pitcher, washed it real good until it shined crystal clear and poured the lemonade in it .

I drew a large homemade sign and Nickey colored it with a rainbow of colors

FOR SALE-LEMONADE (Ice- Cold)
5cents-small
10cents-large

Nickey and I bought a rickety table and two wooden chairs at the Salvation Army store. We set up our lemonade stand in front of our South Bronx apartment building. We made ourselves very visible, as the people passed by,they could not resist but to buy our ice- cold refreshing lemonade. We also bought a tall ceramic black cat bank with green watchful eyes to save our earnings to make our dream real.

Unfortunately, Nicholas died at age 22, and at age 41, I was diagnosed with a rare thyroid cancer, with an unknown prognosis. While I was recovering from a colossal 12 hour neck and chest surgery and 33 high dose radiation treatments I bought two round-trip tickets to San Francisco, California over the phone I loudly whispered to the agent as my vocal cords were damaged. I was so excited about going to California.

Sitting in the middle seat on the plane to San Francisco, I met a pilot named Martin and a grief-stricken nurse, Cheryl. A wonderful conversation ensued and the pilot gave me a monetary gift of $160 to buy dinner and a show for my husband and I (angels in disguise).

The plane finally arrived in California. I stepped off the plane and I heard the song, I Left My Heart In San Francisco (one of my mother's favorite songs) I turned slightly-heart beating rapidly with great anticipation, I see a lemonade stand. With tears rolling down my cheeks, I rush over and buy the $1.50 refreshing cup of lemonade. I look up at the sky and say joyfully,"HERE'S TO OUR DREAM,NICKEY, I LOVE YOU WITH ALL MY HEART."

Barbara Kimbley

I'M GLAD YOU ARE IN MY DASH

I read of a woman who stood to speak
At the funeral of her brother
She referred to the dates on his tombstone
From the beginning...to end.
She noted that first came his birth
And spoke the following date, January 22, 1964 with tears,
But she said what mattered most of all
Was the dash between those years
(1964-1986)
For that dash represents all the time
That he spent alive on earth...
And now only those who loved him
Know what that little line is worth.
For it matters not, how much we own;
The cars...the house...the cash,
What matters is how we live and love
And how we spend our dash.
So think about this long and hard...
Are there things you'd like to change?
For you never know how much time is left,
That can still be rearranged.
If we could just slow down enough
To consider what's true and real,
And always try to understand
The way other people feel.
And be less quick to anger or judge,
and show appreciation more
And love the people in our lives
Like we've never loved before.
If we treat each other with respect,
And more often wear a smile...
Remembering that this special dash
might only last awhile.
So when your eulogy's being read
With your life's actions to rehash...
Would you be proud of the things people say
About how you spent your dash?

UNKNOWN

I read this mass card ,given to me by our dear family friend, Lee P.at Nickey's funeral and believe it in my heart:

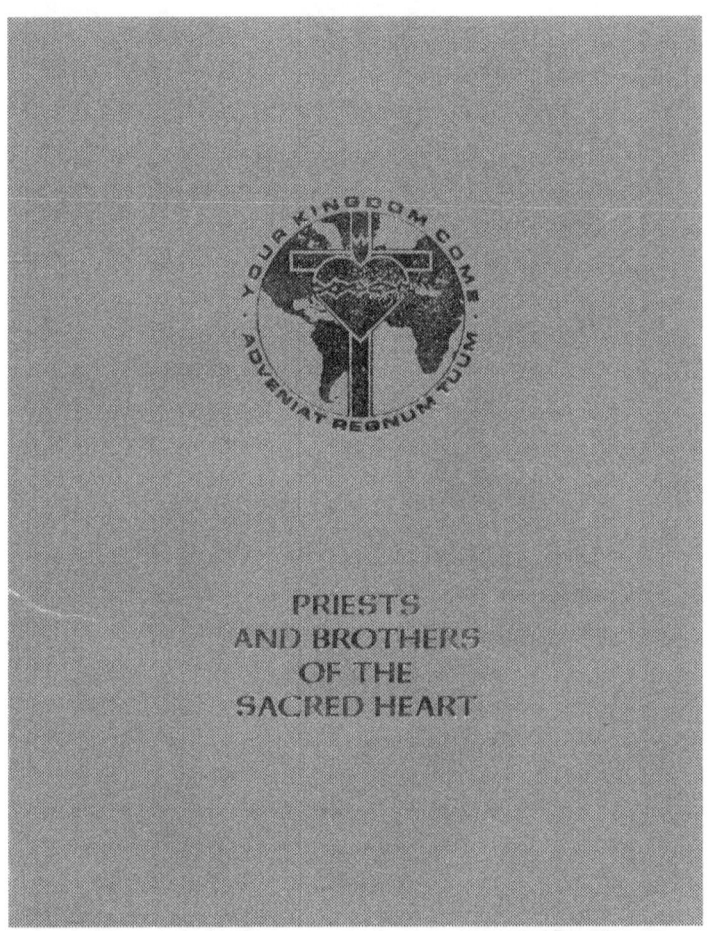

PRIESTS
AND BROTHERS
OF THE
SACRED HEART

Barbara Kimbley

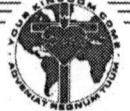

SACRED HEART MEMORIAL

In Memory Of

Nicholas Briggs

The Priests and Brothers of the Sacred Heart
have received a Memorial Gift, together with
the request that the Soul of Your Loved One be
remembered daily in their Masses and Prayers
as long as the Grace of God is needed. May this
thoughtful tribute bring Solace and Consola-
tion to you, as it likewise helps to spread the
Kingdom of God on earth.

Fr. Brian, S.C.J.

Requested by: *Rita Papas*

Priests and Brothers of the Sacred Heart
Sacred Heart Monastery
P.O. Box 900
Hales Corners, WI 53130

SAFELY HOME

I am at home in heaven,dear ones;
Oh,so happy and so bright!
There is perfect joy and beauty
In this everlasting light.

All the pain and grief is over,
Every restless tossing passed;
I am now at peace for ever,
Safely home in Heaven at last.

Did you wonder I so calmly
Trod the valley of the shade?
OH! But Jesus' love illumined
Every dark and fearful glade.

And He came Himself (Angel in the light) to meet me
In that way so hard to tread(thief of the night);
And with Jesus'arm to lean on,
Could I have one doubt or dread?

Then you must not grieve so sorely,
For I love you dearly still:
Try to look beyond earth's shadows,
Pray to trust our Father's Will.

There is work still waiting for you,
So you must not idly stand;
Do it now ,while life remaineth-
You shall rest in Jesus 'land.

When the work is all completed,
He will gently call you Home;
Oh, the rapture of that meeting,
Oh, the joy to see you come!

Barbara Kimbley

To my Readers:
I SAID A PRAYER FOR YOU TODAY-
(My niece, Jennifer gave me this prayer card when
I was diagnosed with Cancer, in 2000)...

I said a prayer for you today
And know God must have heard.
I felt the answer in my heart
Although He spoke not a word.
I didn't ask for wealth or fame
(I knew you wouldn't mind. I asked for priceless
treasures rare)
Of a more lasting kind.
I prayed that He'd be near you
At the start of each new day
To grant you health and blessings fair,
And friends to share your way.
I asked for happiness for you.
In all things great and small
But that you'd know his loving care
I prayed the most of all.

I REMEMBER NICKEY:

Going to school
Eager to learn
Adding and subtracting
Spelling
Reading and writing
Kneeling and praying as a child
Running
Jumping
Pretending to be doctor and patient
          Cowboys and Indians
          Teacher and student
Taking MMs for aspirins with a glass of water
Doing tumblesaults
Riding his first bicycle
Eating pizza at Luigis pizza (South Bronx)
Eating Italian ices-double scoop-lemon, chocolate,
sometimes rainbow
Setting up a lemonade stand with me
Making homemade lemonade
Buying ice—cones -shaved ice from the iceman-grape
and cola
Enjoying Mr. Softee icecream cones
Waiting at the bus-stop to go to work
Enjoying our hot tea or hot chocolate with a buttered
roll every morning before work
Building a snowman
Making snow-angels
Taking long walks with me
Having long talks
Crying
Laughing

Making a family photo album with me
Making a movie log of his favorite movie collection
Taking the learners permit and passing
Buying a little red car with his hard earned money and driving it
Dressing up in a navy blue suit for a night on the town in NY C..-Sardi's for dinner and Barnum and Bailey Circus with our dear friend Lee
Having a beer at Giggles with Elaine
Buying a huge Christmas tree,tying it to the car while rich drove home-we laughed all the way…
Buying me a musical jewelry box for Christmas
First girlfriend
Saying a young woman he dated thought he was just like the actor James Dean-expressions and body language
Baking me a birthday cake from scratch-(sweetheart cake with homemade orange icing)

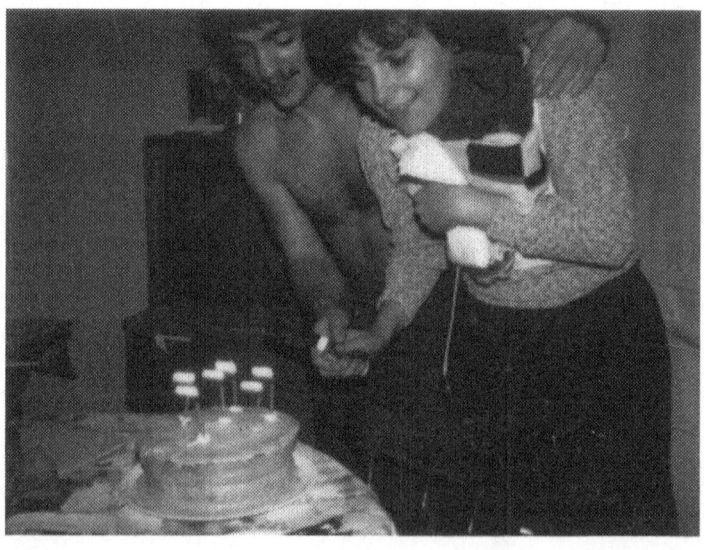

Giving me a surprise party-memorable and treasured event

Flying on a plane(first time flying) to Florida to visit his sister and family

Diving

Swimming

Jones Beach

Singing

Dancing

Praying to God

Holding my hand; being so frightened

Hugging me tight

Dying

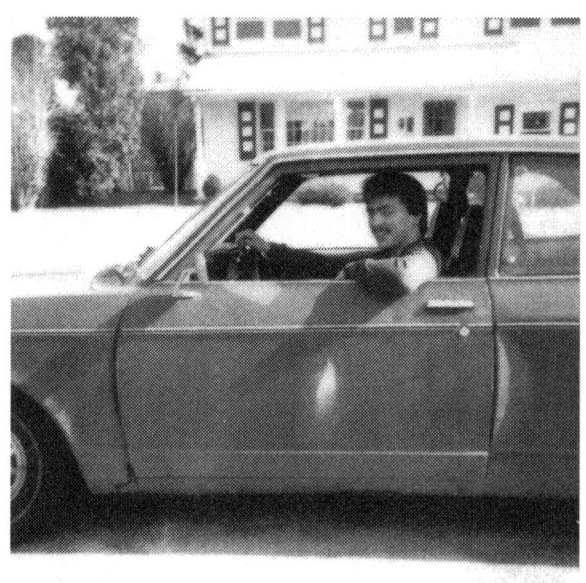

I had a nice time with MY sister Apr-17-1983

From Nichols

Nick's First & Only Car (Little Red)

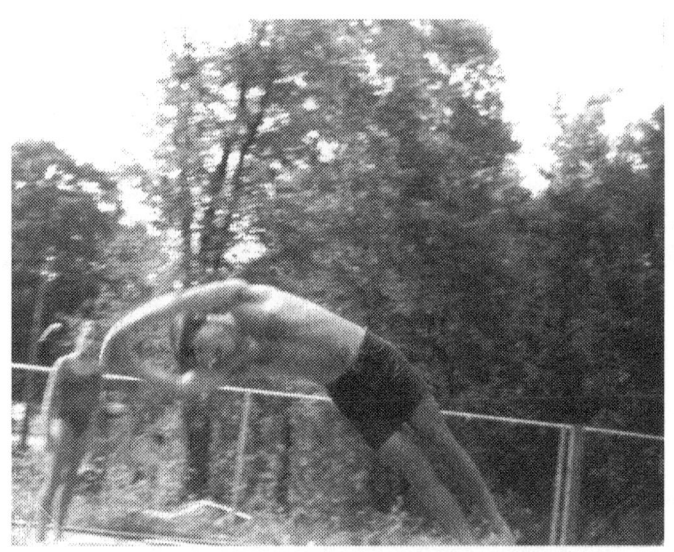

Diving In Aunt Shirley's Pool (Florida N.Y)

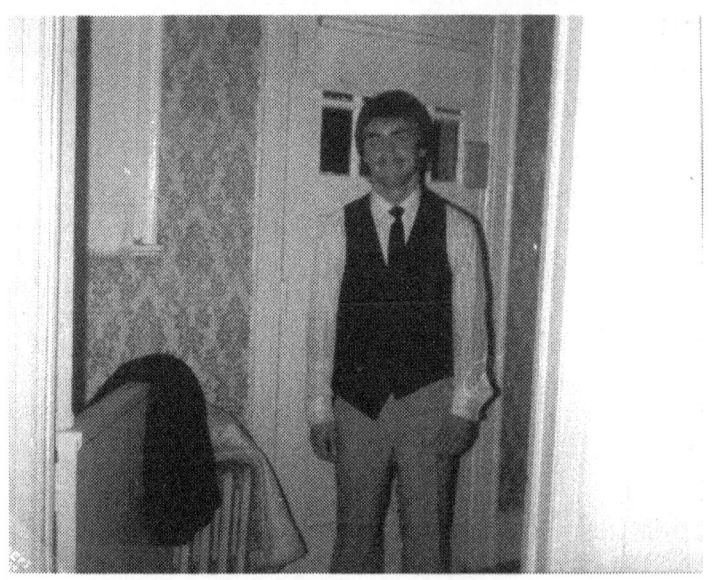

A Night On The Town In The City That Never Sleeps!
With Our Dear Friend Lee P.

Memories-Found this in a prayer book

The sorrow when a loved one dies, goes far beyond the
mind
It penetrates the heart and soul, in anger that is blind
The pain of losing one we love, we think will never heal
So many answers never known, so many questions now
Unreal
But love can heal a grieving soul, in hands held silently
Love can mend a broken heart, when shared so tenderly
Love can find the words we need, to comfort those in
Pain
Love can walk through darkened halls like rainbows in
the rain
Lord teach us to walk down our pathway today
The way that You walked to the garden to pray
With faith and the knowledge of what lay ahead
Yet so humbly fearlessly onward you tread
Lord teach us to pray the way you prayed
Unceasingly faithfully honestly made
For those of us here that have gathered in love
We know that our loved one is with You above
For their soul will live eternally
And so in our minds their memories
Their love, laughter, and our tears
Precious moments,
Always near.
Amen.

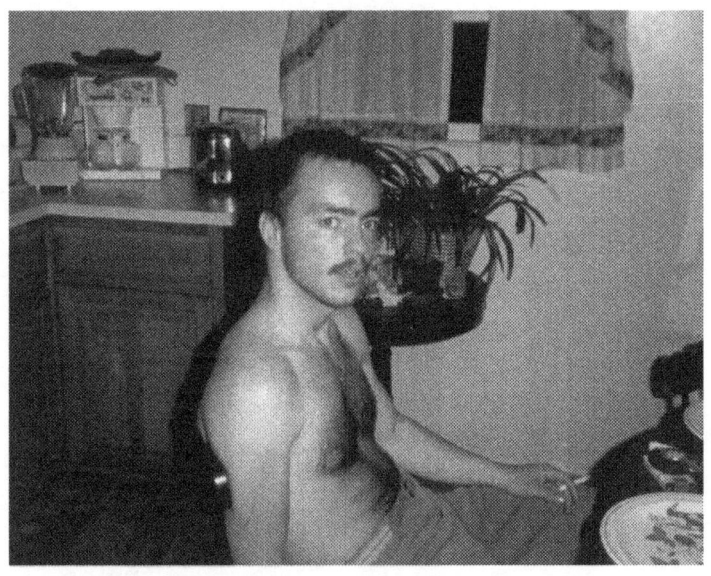

Nickey's final days at home before being readmitted
into the hospital 1986 Levittown NY

"We have loved them during life; let us not abandon them until we have conducted them by our prayers into the house of the Lord."   St. AMBROSE

**Of Your Charity Pray For
The Repose of the Soul of**

NICHOLAS MICHAEL BRIGGS
**Born January 22, 1964
Died November 29, 1986**

"O Lord support us all the day long of this troublous life, until the shadows lengthen and evening comes and the busy world is hushed and the fever of life is over and our work is done. Then of Thy great mercy grant us a safe lodging and a Holy rest and peace at the last, through Jesus Christ, our Lord. Amen."

—Cardinal Newman

"I am the resurrection and the life, he who believes in me even if he die, shall live..."

———

Alba 27 **THOMAS F. DALTON**
Funeral Home

A Letter I wrote to my brother in heaven ....

Sunday 1/4/87

Dearest Nicholas,My Brother:

I love you & miss you.
It's very quiet around here without you.
Nicholas, what do you think about the house?
Is it for me or should I wait for a better opportunity?
Nicholas give me an answer-
Nicholas-what's it like in heaven??
Is it beautiful and peaceful?
I look up at the sky and I see so much beauty.
I wonder if it's the same where you are-
Nicholas watch over me always if you can-
Can you hear me when I talk to you?
Do you want a cup of tea?
Actually, you'd be sleeping by now-
Thanks for all your equipment-we're enjoying it-
especially the tape you made last year-
It's so much like you-so natural.
Nick, I can't believe you died-
Give a hug to Rommie for me and Grandma and Papa,
Paul, Mike , Aunt Pearl,Agnes, Mike and Uncle Walter,
and anyone else I might know
Gladys Reilly,Lester, Kim(Richie's father) and Lenny
(Richie's brother)

Love Your sister, Barbara

About the Book:

Read this heart-breaking and yet heart-warming true story about my brother, Nickey who lived fast and died young at age 22. He was born in the South Bronx, lived on the lower East side streets, park benches and alleyways of Spanish Harlem, as a child. As a young adult, he lived in Wantagh and Levittown, Long Island with his sister .I was inspired to write this book because my brother was precious to me and I want to share his story. If you read my brother's short life story and walk away with knowledge about A.I.D.S. and warmth in your heart then my brother, Nickey will live on in memory and his young life will be valued not only by me, but by many worldwide.

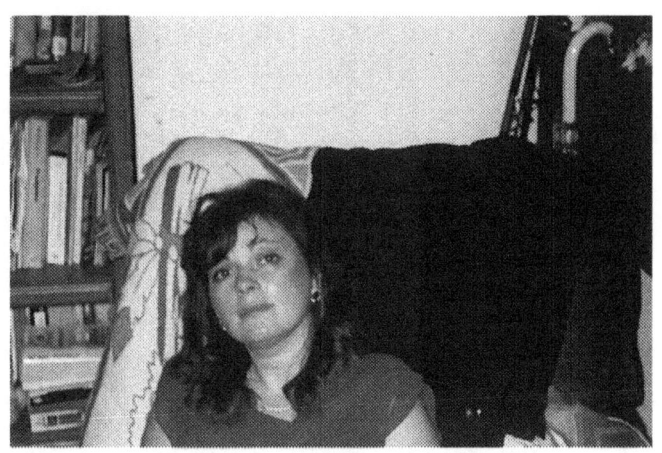

About the Author:

Barbara Kimbley resides in sunny Florida moving here in 1989 from Long Island, NY Born September 22,1958 in Manhattan, NY She is medically retired from a wonderful and rewarding career with J. C. Penneys. April 2000, she was diagnosed with a rare thyroid cancer. She is not in remission, just stable and guarded. She started writing about her cancer journey then decided to write about her brother's short life story first. She is determined, persistent, resilient, diplomatic and has a strong will to live. Married to a devoted and loving husband, Richie (teenage sweethearts with a 31 year relationship). Her grown son, Rich Jr. is intelligent and charismatic, works in Public Relations and her wonderful daughter-in-law is a graphic designer. She has an older sister, Lana who she admires for overcoming her tragedies and struggles in life with dedication and fortitude. She has a passion for people, loves to travel, and enjoys playing Scrabble and reading self-help books. Among her many roles, she is a customer service manager, retail trainer, model, wife, mother, daughter, sister and broadcast journalist. She plans to share her personal cancer journey with you, her readers, in the near future.

J. C. Penneys associate, Virginia Petrie gave me this poem when Nickey died.

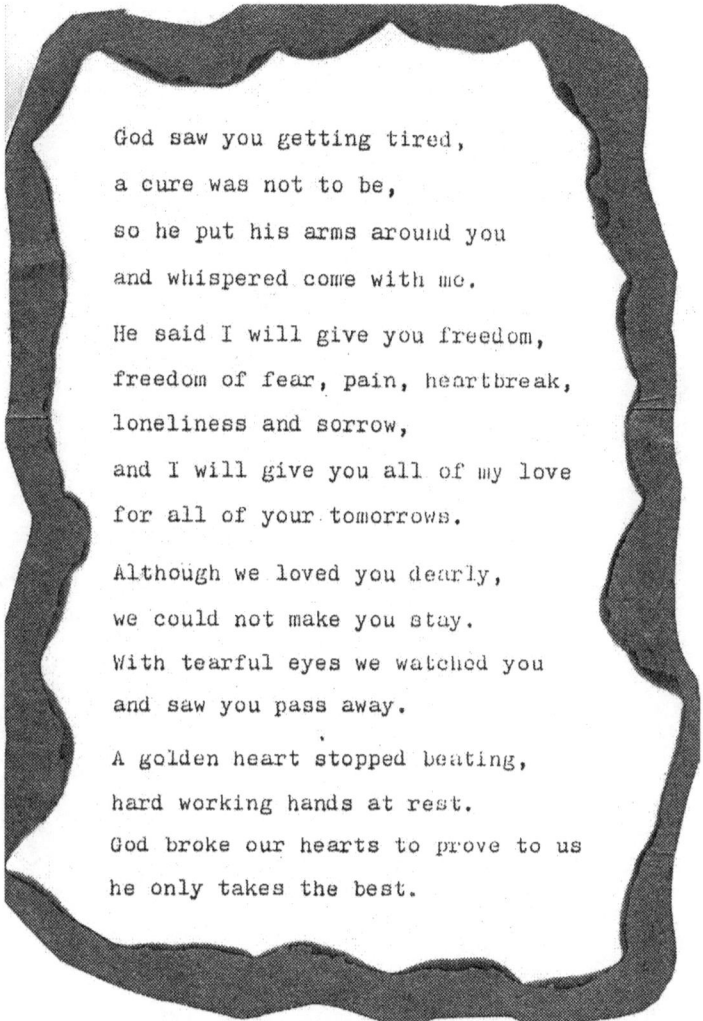

God saw you getting tired,
a cure was not to be,
so he put his arms around you
and whispered come with me.

He said I will give you freedom,
freedom of fear, pain, heartbreak,
loneliness and sorrow,
and I will give you all of my love
for all of your tomorrows.

Although we loved you dearly,
we could not make you stay.
With tearful eyes we watched you
and saw you pass away.

A golden heart stopped beating,
hard working hands at rest.
God broke our hearts to prove to us
he only takes the best.

Nickey you will always have a special place in our hearts.
Love your sister, Barbara